Management of Peripheral Arterial Disease

Medical, Surgical and Interventional Aspects

ReMEDICA State of the Art series
ISSN 1472-4626

Also available
Management of Atherosclerotic Carotid Disease

Forthcoming titles
Management of Inflammatory Bowel Disease
Management of Rheumatoid Arthritis

Published by ReMEDICA Publishing Limited
32-38 Osnaburgh Street, London, NW1 3ND, UK

Tel: +44 207 388 7677
Fax: +44 207 388 7678
Email: books@remedica.com
www.remedica.com

© 2000 ReMEDICA Publishing Limited
Publication date October 2000

ISBN 1 901346 14 5
British Library Cataloguing-in-Publication Data
A catalogue record for this book is available from the British Library.

Management of Peripheral Arterial Disease

Medical, Surgical and Interventional Aspects

Editor
Mark Creager
Brigham and Women's Hospital
Boston, MA, USA

ReMEDICA*PUBLISHING*

Contributors

Editor

Mark A Creager
Associate Professor of Medicine
Harvard Medical School
Cardiovascular Division
Director, Vascular Center
Brigham and Women's Hospital
75 Francis Street
Boston, MA 02115, USA

Authors

Joshua Beckman
Instructor in Medicine
Harvard Medical School
Cardiovascular Division
Brigham and Women's Hospital
75 Francis Street
Boston, MA 02115, USA

Warner Bundens
Department of Surgery
University of California, San Diego
9500 Gilman Drive
La Jolla, CA 92093, USA

Mark A Creager
Associate Professor of Medicine
Harvard Medical School
Cardiovascular Division
Director, Vascular Center
Brigham and Women's Hospital
75 Francis Street
Boston, MA 02115, USA

Michael H Criqui
Professor and Vice Chair,
Dept of Family and Preventive Medicine
Professor, Dept of Medicine
Director, Preventive Cardiology Academic Award
University of California, San Diego
9500 Gilman Drive
La Jolla, CA 92093, USA

Mandeep Dhadly
Division of Vascular Medicine
St Elizabeth's Medical Center
736 Cambridge Street
Boston, MA 02135, USA

Beatrice Golomb
Department of Medicine
University of California, San Diego
9500 Gilman Drive
La Jolla, CA 92093, USA

William R Hiatt
Novartis Professor of Cardiovascular
Research
Section of Vascular Medicine
University of Colorado
Health Sciences Center
Executive Director
Colorado Prevention Center
789 Sherman Street
Suite 200
Denver, CO 80203, USA

Michael Jaff
Medical Director,
Center for Vascular Care
Co-Director,
Vascular Diagnostic Laboratory
Washington Hospital Center
Washington, DC 20010, USA

Michael Lepore
Alton Ochsner Medical Foundation
Tulane University School of Medicine
New Orleans, LA 70121, USA

Samuel Money
Head, Division of Vascular Surgery
Alton Ochsner Medical Foundation
Tulane University School of Medicine
New Orleans, LA 70121, USA

Kenneth Rosenfield
Assistant Professor of Medicine
Division of Vascular Medicine
St Elizabeth's Medical Center
736 Cambridge Street
Boston, MA 02135, USA

Preface

Peripheral arterial disease is a clinical manifestation of atherosclerosis. The term is often used in reference to non-coronary atherosclerosis, particularly that affecting the lower and upper limbs. Recent advances in vascular biology and new discoveries in the biomedical arena have increased our ability to treat peripheral arterial disease and to reduce the disabling and fatal consequences of atherosclerosis.

This book is a focused, yet comprehensive, review of peripheral arterial disease. It includes current information that should be particularly useful to the practicing physician.

Chapter 1 provides background material on the epidemiology of peripheral arterial disease, emphasizing its prevalence and its association with other cardiovascular diseases.

Chapter 2 builds upon this information whilst focusing on the importance of risk factor modification and antiplatelet therapy in reduction of adverse cardiovascular events.

Chapter 3 discusses the pathophysiology of peripheral arterial disease, in particular how it applies to the development of symptoms and disability. As such, it sets the stage for therapeutic interventions, which are discussed in the following chapters.

Chapter 4 focuses on pharmacotherapy. Until recently, few—if any—drugs had been identified as effective in improving symptoms of peripheral arterial disease, despite great efforts by the pharmaceutical industry. The efficacy of current agents as well as the potential utility of newer drugs is discussed.

Chapter 5 reviews contemporary surgical approaches for revascularizing patients with peripheral arterial disease, particularly those with disabling claudication or critical limb ischemia. Though familiar to most vascular surgeons, the information contained in this chapter will provide other physicians with an insight into the rationale, technical considerations and outcome of patients treated with vascular reconstructive surgery.

Chapter 6 describes the exciting developments in treatment of patients using catheter-based, endovascular interventions. Technical considerations for endovascular intervention apply to a wide range of vascular problems, and this chapter discusses not only peripheral arterial disease of the limbs but also the application of catheter-based therapy in brachiocephalic and renal arteries.

Patients with vascular disease constitute an increasing proportion of physicians' practices. I believe this book will raise awareness of peripheral arterial disease and provide the physician with the cognitive tools necessary for treating patients with this disorder.

Mark A Creager, M.D.
Brigham and Women's Hospital, Boston, MA, USA

October 2000

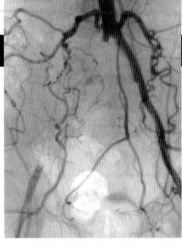

ReMEDICA_PUBLISHING_

Management of Peripheral Arterial Disease

chapter one

Epidemiology

Beatrice Golomb, Michael Criqui and Warner Bundens

Introduction

Peripheral arterial disease (PAD) is generally defined as partial or complete obstruction of one or more arteries, usually of the pelvis or lower limbs, caused by atherosclerosis. It may be asymptomatic, or manifested by symptoms of compromised blood flow with exercise or, in severe cases, at rest. Symptomatic PAD, particularly claudication (pain in the lower extremities typically brought on by walking and relieved by rest), has been estimated to reduce quality of life in at least 2 million individuals in the USA [1], and figures for prevalence of asymptomatic disease are several fold higher.

Estimates of PAD incidence and prevalence are of more than academic interest. Although comparatively modest numbers of deaths are directly ascribed to PAD, it has important morbidity and mortality implications. Symptomatic disease directly affects functional capacity and quality of life by inducing pain and restricting ambulation. Asymptomatic disease is also important, as it may presage future risk of compromised ambulation, lower extremity ulcers and the need for vascular surgery or amputation. Moreover, asymptomatic, as well as symptomatic, disease is a consistent and powerful independent predictor of coronary artery disease (CAD) and cerebrovascular disease events and mortality.

PAD, which is strongly age-dependent, is increasing in prevalence as the population ages. Data from subjects in the Framingham study, one of the few studies to assess incidence by age, found that onset of symptomatic disease, defined by intermittent claudication (IC), increased 10-fold in men from age 30–44 to 65–74 (with an incidence of 6/10,000 in the former group and 61/10,000 in the latter). In women, onset rose almost 20-fold from the younger to older age-groups (3/10,000 rising to 54/10,000) [2].

Other studies have found 5-year incidence rates of 7.5% in 55–74 year old men and women [3]. However, the incidence data from these two studies underestimate clinically relevant PAD, as they are confined to symptomatic disease.

Prevalence data show clearly that symptomatic disease represents a modest fraction of all clinically important PAD. Prevalence rates increase when more liberal criteria for symptomatic disease are employed (including atypical symptoms as well as those meeting "Rose criteria"), and increase further when PAD is defined by objective non-invasive criteria, typically an ankle-brachial index, or ABI (ratio of lower to upper extremity blood pressure values, signifying lower systolic blood pressure at the ankle compared to that at the arm) of ≤ 0.9. Reported IC prevalence has varied from 1.6–12%, while rates of non-invasively defined disease have ranged from 3.8–33% [4–16]. Estimates are strongly dependent on the age of the examined population, as illustrated in Table 1 (data from Rotterdam and San Diego) [7,12]; within-population prevalence rates rise markedly with increasing age, both for IC and for non-invasively defined disease. Note that although these are two completely separate populations in different countries, and the PAD assessment was somewhat different, the age-specific rates of non-invasively-defined PAD and IC are similar. Also, note that in both populations only a minority of PAD patients have IC.

> ABI = the ratio of ankle to arm systolic blood pressure, with an abnormal ratio typically defined as ≤ 0.90

Incidentally, there is a small positive association of ABI with height [10,17,18], leading to higher average ABI in younger men compared to women. However, men experience accelerated decrement in ABI, consistent with their greater risk of atherosclerosis. Thus, studies confined to older populations or those using lower ABI cut-offs typically show a male preponderance, although the discrepancy is smaller than that seen with CAD.

It is important to note that the presence of IC is not only an insensitive marker of PAD, but also may not have good predictive value for PAD defined by non-invasive objective measures. In a study conducted in Rotterdam, a mere

Table 1. Prevalence estimates of peripheral arterial disease and intermittent claudication by age: Rotterdam study and San Diego population study.

Age	Rotterdam [12]*		Age	San Diego Population Study [7]**	
	PAD by ABI <0.9, %	IC, %		PAD by NI tests, %**	IC, %
40–45			40–45		
45–49			45–49	2.5	0.0
50–54			50–54		
55–59	9	1.0	55–59		
60–64	11	1.2	60–64	8.3	2.4
65–69	15	1.7	65–69		
70–74	17	2.3	70–74	18.8	2.7
75–79	23	3.2	75–79		
80–84	40	4.0	80–84		
85–89	57	5.0	85–89		

*Prevalence figures for Rotterdam Study are estimates derived from figure. Elderly community based cohort from Rotterdam (5450 males and females) age >55; male age 69 ± 9, female 72 ± 10.

**Population study of 624 males and females (38–82 year olds). Non-invasive (NI) tests = segmental blood pressure above-knee, below-knee, at ankle, at toe divided by brachial pressure and three measures of flow velocity in each of the femoral and posterior tibial arteries.

6.3% of those with ABI<0.9 had classic IC (8.7% of men and 4.9% of women). Moreover, only 69% of those with IC had ABI<0.9 [12], reflecting, at best, a moderate positive predictive value of IC for PAD. Similarly, in the Edinburgh artery study, only 63% of those with IC had ABI<0.9 [10].

Formal evaluation of the sensitivity, specificity and positive and negative predictive value (PPV and NPV) of IC for non-invasively defined disease was undertaken in 624 subjects in the San Diego population study, and showed poor sensitivity but somewhat higher specificity. Rose claudication had a sensitivity of 9.2%, specificity of 99%, PPV of 55% and NPV of 90% [19]. When Rose or possible claudication was evaluated, sensitivity rose to 20% and specificity declined to 96%, with 38% PPV and 90% NPV. Naturally, the sensitivity of IC as a marker for PAD decreases, and the specificity increases, as more restrictive non-invasive criteria are chosen against which to compare IC. If claudication assessment is performed, the San Diego Claudication Questionnaire (see Appendix 1 on page 14) should be preferred over the Rose and Edinburgh questionnaires, because it entails separate analysis for each leg [20]. This strategy, among other benefits, prevents falsely classifying subjects who experience claudication in one leg but non-ischemic pain in the contralateral limb as free of claudication; the presence of the non-ischemic pain would falsely disqualify them from a diagnosis of claudication in instruments that fail to rate each leg separately.

Peripheral pulse evaluation is a traditional clinical examination for PAD. However, neither peripheral pulses nor femoral bruits have adequate sensitivity, specificity or predictive value to be reliable markers for PAD [19].

Co-prevalence of PAD with cardiovascular disease

Populations with CAD and cerebrovascular disease have markedly increased prevalence of PAD. Moreover, those with PAD have markedly increased prevalence of CAD and cerebrovascular disease.

PAD in those with CAD and cerebrovascular disease

In a San Diego population study, 32% of men with clinical cardiovascular disease, including CAD and cerebrovascular disease, also had PAD, compared to 13% of men without cardiovascular disease; 25% of women with cardiovascular disease, versus 11% of women without, met non-invasive criteria for PAD. This signifies a 2–3 fold excess [21]. A Saudi study of patients aged 50–80 (mean 59) showed a PAD prevalence of 21% in those with ischemic heart disease, contrasted with 4% in controls without heart disease, renal disease or diabetes, suggesting up to a 5-fold increase [22].

CAD and cerebrovascular disease in those with PAD

In a San Diego population study of subjects aged 38–82, clinical cardiovascular disease (CAD or cerebrovascular disease) was present in 29% of men with non-invasively defined PAD, compared to 12% of men without PAD; 21% of women with PAD also had cardiovascular disease, compared to 9% of women without cardiovascular disease [21]. This indicates a 2–3 fold excess of cardiovascular disease in the presence of PAD. A cross-sectional study of a stratified sample of patients from 18 general practice clinics, with a PAD prevalence of 6.9%, showed a 3–4 fold excess of cardiovascular disease in those with non-invasively defined PAD (ABI<0.95) [6].

Examining CAD more specifically, a review by Dormandy found prevalence rates of CAD in PAD patients ranging from a low of 19% (clinical history + electrocardiogram [ECG]) to a mid-range of 62% (stress ECG or dipyridamole-stress thallium) to a high of 90% (angiography) (Table 2); the differences are substantially the consequence of differences in the sensitivity of criteria for CAD. Table 2 is modified from Dormandy, 1989 [23], updated to include more recent references [24,25].

PAD may be a particularly potent predictor of cerebrovascular disease, which has been reported to occur in approximately a quarter of PAD patients. In the Dormandy review, PAD was associated with carotid stenosis on Doppler imaging, and cerebrovascular events, with the prevalence of cerebrovascular disease in PAD again directly related to the sensitivity of cerebrovascular disease assessment [23]. (Thus, for instance, stroke history is far less common than carotid stenosis gauged by non-invasive imaging.) Table 3 is modified from Dormandy, 1989 [23], and updated [25-28]. PAD may be an even stronger predictor of intercurrent cerebrovascular disease than traditional risk-signifying markers such as carotid bruits. Routine carotid duplex scans were performed in Chinese subjects and showed that those with PAD had the highest prevalence of significant (>70% diameter) carotid stenosis (24.5%) when compared to patients with CAD (11%), carotid bruits (10%) or aortic aneurysms (9%), and with normal controls (0%; p<0.001) [28].

Subjects from San Diego (203) underwent concomitant non-invasive testing for suspicion of PAD and non-invasive carotid duplex imaging. This showed a modest but significant correlation between severity of PAD and severity of carotid disease (defined using three measures from each carotid system: internal, external and common carotids) in a population with a high prevalence of both [29]. Four non-invasive measures from each leg, including the ABI, were used to devise an aggregate standard PAD score.

Table 2. Coronary artery disease prevalence in patients presenting with peripheral arterial disease (selected studies*).

Citation	n	CAD assessment	% with CAD
Begg (1962)	198	Clinical history + ECG	19
Szilagyi (1979)	531	Clinical history + ECG	39
Malone (1977)	180	Clinical history + ECG	58
DeWeese (1977)	103	Clinical history + ECG	34
Hughson (1978)	160	Clinical history + ECG	36
Crawford (1981)	949	Clinical history + ECG	38
Hertzer (1981)	256	Clinical history + ECG	47
Szilagyi (1986)	1748	Uncertain	47
Mendelson (1998)	213	Clinical history + ECG	62
Vecht (1982)	100	Modified treadmill stress ECG	62
Brewster (1985)	54	Dipyridamole-stress thallium	63
Valentine (1994)	59	Angiography	71
Hertzer (1984)	381	Angiography	90

*Adapted with permission from Dormandy 1989 [23], and updated [24,25] (see Dormandy [23] for remaining full citations).

This showed a correlation of r = 0.23 (p<0.001) to number of diseased carotids (>50% diameter stenosis), and a correlation of r = 0.23 to average carotid occlusive disease score; these correlations were slightly reduced, to 0.21 (p = 0.043) and 0.17 (p = 0.092), after exclusion of approximately 50% of subjects who had undergone surgical intervention of either carotids or lower extremities.

Morbidity and mortality implications

In light of the high co-prevalence of cerebrovascular disease and CAD in patients with PAD, as well as the overlap in measured and unmeasured risk factors that may signify increased future risk of cerebrovascular disease and CAD even if cardiovascular disease is not presently identified, it should come as no surprise that the presence of PAD predicts future cardiovascular and cerebrovascular morbidity and mortality, and all-cause mortality. Most existing evidence suggests that PAD signifies independent

Table 3. Cerebrovascular disease prevalence in patients presenting with peripheral arterial disease (selected studies*).

Citation	n	Cerebrovascular disease assessment	% with cerebrovascular disease
Begg (1962)	198	Clinical history	0.5
DeWeese (1977)	103	Clinical history	4
Szilagyi (1979)	531	Clinical history ± angiography	13
Hughson (1978)	54	Clinical history	15
Szilagyi (1986)	1748	Uncertain	19
Cheng (1999)	186	Duplex stenosis >70%	25
Alexandrova (1996)	373	Duplex stenosis >60%	25
Mendelson (1998)	34	Clinical history	35
Malone (1977)	180	Clinical history and clinical exam (includes cervical bruit)	45
Turnipseed (1980)	160	Cervical bruit	44
Alexandrova (1996)	373	Duplex 30% stenosis	57
Turnipseed (1980)	160	Non-invasive tests (doppler)	52
Cheng (1999)	186	Duplex >30% stenosis	67

*Adapted with permission from Dormandy 1989 [23], and updated [25-27] (see Dormandy [23] for remaining full citations).

increased risk for CAD and cerebrovascular disease, in addition to that conferred by intercurrent major coronary risk factors, serving as a proxy for the actions of unmeasured or unadjusted risk factors, and as a marker of ongoing disease. Moreover, PAD has prognostic implications for those with, and without, identified CAD and cerebrovascular disease.

Implications for PAD morbidity and mortality

In a study from Edinburgh, among those with IC at baseline, 8.2% underwent vascular surgery or amputation and 1.4% developed leg ulceration after 5 years [3]. In another study, among IC patients without other clinical indicators, 7.5% progressed to rest pain, ulcers or gangrene in the first year, with 2.2% converting annually thereafter, over a 6.5-year follow-up [30]. Although PAD complications are strikingly higher in those with baseline PAD than those without, they are nonetheless overshadowed in PAD patients by other atherosclerotic events. Thus, in subjects with IC in the Framingham study, 50% of deaths were from CAD, 10% from cerebrovascular disease, and 13% from "other vascular" causes, including more direct PAD causes [2,23].

Implications for CAD morbidity and mortality

PAD, by any of an assortment of criteria, is associated with increased risk of CAD. New angina, non-fatal myocardial infarction (MI), congestive heart failure (CHF) and fatal MI or CAD death are all increased [3,4,8,12,31,32]. Whether PAD is symptomatic or asymptomatic, studies have shown a 20–40% increased risk for nonfatal MI [3], a 60% increased risk of progression to CHF even after multivariate adjustment (in those without prior identified cardiovascular disease) [8], and a 90–500% increased risk of fatal MI and CAD death [3,4,13,32]. The greatest increase in risk was seen in a population-based study with a somewhat more stringent PAD definition (e.g. ABI cutoff <0.8) and 10-year follow-up. Although full multivariate adjustment was performed, data from this study suggested that limited adjustment, e.g. for age and sex, yields risk ratios similar to those obtained with full adjustment [32]. Data from this population study confirm a relationship between PAD severity and CAD mortality risk. Among men, 11% of those with normal vascular supply in this population (age 38–82, mean 66) experienced CAD death on a 10-year follow-up, compared to nearly 40% of those with moderate PAD (defined as ABI between 0.6 and 0.9) and over 60% of those with severe PAD (ABI<0.6); mortality figures for women paralleled those for men but were just over half the rate for each group [33].

Implications for cerebrovascular disease morbidity and mortality

PAD predicts increased cerebrovascular disease outcomes in some studies. Thus, ABI<0.9 was associated with increased nonfatal stroke (although not fatal stroke) in one study [29], while, in another, increasing PAD severity was correlated with the combined outcome of transient ischemic attack (TIA) and definite and possible stroke [3]. An analysis of Spanish subjects showed that PAD was correlated not only with ischemic stroke, but also with hemorrhagic stroke — indeed, the risk ratio for the latter was rather higher than that for ischemic stroke [34]. PAD has been linked to worse outcome in patients who experience a stroke [35].

Implications for overall cardiovascular disease morbidity and mortality

Since PAD is linked to increased CAD and cerebrovascular disease events and mortality, it would be expected to be linked to increased overall cardiovascular morbidity and mortality. Indeed, both combined cardiovascular disease morbidity and mortality, and cardiovascular disease mortality per se, are increased in those with PAD, by all PAD definitions employed, with risk ratios of the order of 2–6 [3,4,8,13,31,32]. More stringent PAD criteria (signifying more severe PAD) are again linked to greater risk ratios; thus, the San Diego study [33] showed higher risk ratios than studies using ABI<0.9.

Implications for overall mortality

While some major risk factors for cardiovascular disease predict cardiovascular disease mortality but not overall mortality, PAD is a powerful predictor not only of cardiovascular disease outcomes but also of overall mortality — in men, women, elderly subjects, community cohorts and among other groups, with 50–400% increases in risk [3,4,8,13,30–32,36,37]. A San Diego population-based study showed that, once again, PAD severity is linked to the magnitude of increased risk, with mortalities of 15% in normal subjects, 45% in patients with asymptomatic PAD and 75% in those with severe symptomatic PAD in a 10-year follow-up [32] (Figure 1). Another study, using non-invasive criteria exclusively, found 10-year mortalities of approximately 20% in those with an ABI>0.85, 50% in those with an ABI of 0.4–0.85 and 70% in those with an ABI<0.4 [36] (Figure 2). A study in PAD patients again found that lower values of ABI were associated with progressively greater total mortality [38] (Figure 3). The striking similarity of the survival curves in Figures 1, 2 and 3, based on these three distinct populations, further underscores the point that greater PAD severity predicts greater risk of all-cause mortality.

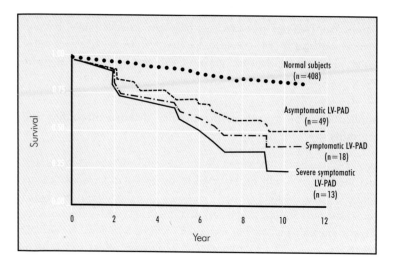

Figure 1. Mortality in patients with large vessel (LV) peripheral arterial disease (PAD).

Criqui MH, Langer RD, Fronek A et al. Mortality over a period of 10 years in patients with peripheral arterial disease. N Engl J Med 1992;326:381-6.

PAD has also been shown to predict increased mortality in specialized groups of patients such as those with acute MI [39] and those undergoing coronary artery bypass grafting (CABG) [40-42]; in the latter group, both in-hospital survival and longer term mortality in those who survive to discharge are predicted by PAD.

The increased risk of CAD mortality, cerebrovascular disease morbidity and mortality, total cardiovascular disease mortality and overall mortality associated with non-invasively defined PAD is illustrated in Table 4, which presents risk ratios and 95% confidence intervals (adjusted for multiple covariates) for these outcomes, using 10–year follow-up data from the San Diego population-based study [32,43].

Summary

PAD is a sometimes asymptomatic, sometimes painful, condition of the lower extremities that increases sharply in prominence with age, becoming common

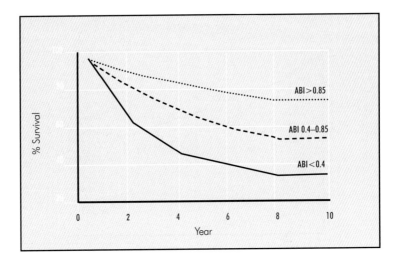

Figure 2. Survival according to ankle-brachial index (ABI).

McKenna M, Wolfson S, Kuller L. The ratio of ankle and arm arterial pressure as an independent predictor of mortality. Atherosclerosis 1991;87:119-28.

among the elderly. Thus, it is of escalating concern as the population ages. Because of shared risk factors for PAD, CAD and cerebrovascular disease, and because of the shared status of these conditions as exemplars of atherosclerotic disease, a high prevalence of co-morbid CAD and cerebrovascular disease is seen in those with PAD. Moreover, PAD is a strong predictor of future CAD and cerebrovascular disease morbidity and mortality, whether or not prior CAD and/or cerebrovascular disease have been diagnosed.

Implications

Because PAD strongly predicts increased risk of CAD and cerebrovascular disease morbidity and mortality, it merits increased consideration in risk assessment for cardiovascular disease and consequently in determining vigor of preventive treatments. Increasing emphasis has been given to the use of risk estimates for cardiovascular disease in determining aggressiveness of preventive treatment [44,45], yet, despite the potency of PAD as a risk predictor, assessment of PAD has not been prominent in published

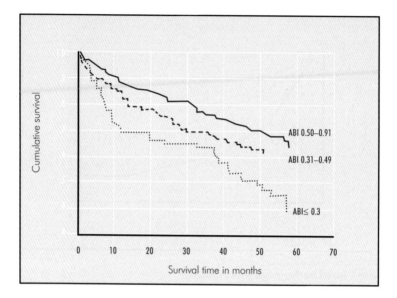

Figure 3. Survival stratified by ankle-brachial index (ABI).

McDermott MM, Feinglass J, Slavensky R et al. The ankle-brachial index as a predictor of survival in patients with peripheral vascular disease. J Gen Intern Med 1994;9:445-9.

risk factor analyses. Moreover, although PAD may be an even stronger predictor of survival in CAD patients than is prior MI, those with CAD are likely to receive more intensive treatment and advice regarding lifestyle factors than those with PAD [39,46,47]. To some degree this may reflect the lesser attention that has been given to PAD, and the consequent lesser body of evidence regarding morbidity and mortality benefits of treatment in those with PAD. Furthermore, the presence and severity of PAD appears to be assessed less systematically than other atherosclerotic conditions. Increased research attention should be accorded to this powerful prognostic factor.

PAD serves as a strong but under-recognized independent predictor of cardiovascular disease risk — or, alternatively conceptualized, as a predictor of the combined impact of unmeasured risk factors and ongoing disease processes. Since cardiovascular disease risk

Table 4. Prediction of coronary artery disease, cerebrovascular disease, cardiovascular disease and overall mortality by peripheral arterial disease.

		Risk ratio	95% confidence intervals
CAD mortality	All	6.6**	2.9–14.9
	No prior cardiovascular disease	4.3**	1.4–2.8
Cerebrovascular disease[†]	Male	3.3*	1.1–9.3
	Female	9.0**	2.3–35.7
Cardiovascular disease mortality	All	5.9***	3.0–11.4
	No prior cardiovascular disease	6.3***	2.6–15.0
Overall mortality	All	3.1***	1.9–4.9
	No prior cardiovascular disease	3.1***	1.8–5.3

*p<0.05; **p<0.01; ***p<0.001

† Includes morbidity and mortality

San Diego Population Study (n = 624, age 38–82, community and employed cohort, 10–year follow-up). PAD defined by segmental blood pressure and flow velocity by Doppler. Risk ratios adjusted for age, body mass index (BMI), cigarettes/day, fasting glucose, log plasma triglycerides, LDL-C, HDL-C and systolic blood pressure [32,43].

assessment is increasingly invoked to guide the fervor of cardiovascular disease preventive treatment efforts [45,48], and PAD powerfully contributes to risk, the presence and severity of PAD should be assessed and incorporated in cardiovascular disease risk analysis. Clearly, this requires increased education of physicians regarding the potent prognostic implications of PAD.

APPENDIX 1

SAN DIEGO CLAUDICATION QUESTIONNAIRE
(INTERVIEWER ADMINISTERED VERSION)

			Right	Left
1) Do you get pain or discomfort in either leg or either buttock on walking? (If no, stop)	No	1	2
	Yes	2	2
2) Does this pain ever begin when you are standing still or sitting?	No	1	1
	Yes	2	2
3) In what part of the leg or buttock do you feel it?			
a) Pain includes calf/calves	No	1	1
	Yes	2	2
b) Pain includes thigh/thighs	No	1	1
	Yes	2	2
c) Pain includes buttock/buttocks	No	1	1
	Yes	2	2
4) Do you get it when you walk uphill or hurry?	No	1	1
	Yes	2	2
	Never walks uphill/hurries..	3	
5) Do you get it when you walk at an ordinary pace on the level?	No	1	1
	Yes	2	2
6) Does the pain ever disappear while you are walking?	No	1	1
	Yes	2	2
7) What do you do if you get it when you are walking?	Stop or slow down	1	1
	Continue on	2	2
8) What happens to it if you stand still? (if unchanged, stop)	Lessened or relieved	1	1
	Unchanged	2	2
9) How soon?	10 min or less	1	1
	More than 10 min	2	2

1) **No pain** – 1 = 1
2) **Pain at rest** – 1 = 2 and 2 = 2
3) **Non-calf** – 1 = 2 and 2 = 1 and 3a = 1 and 3b = 2 or 3c = 2
4) **Non-Rose calf** – 1 = 2 and 2 = 1 and 3a = 2, and not Rose
5) **Rose** – 1 = 2 and 2 = 1 and 3a = 2 and 4 = 2 or 3 (and if 4 = 3, then 5 = 2), and 6 = 1 and 7 = 1 and 8 = 1 and 9 = 1

APPENDIX 1

SAN DIEGO CLAUDICATION QUESTIONNAIRE
(SELF-ADMINISTERED VERSION)

Circle Answer

1) Do you get pain or discomfort in either leg or either buttock on walking?
(If no, stop)

Right leg	Yes	No
Left leg	Yes	No

2) Does this pain ever begin when you are standing still or sitting?

Right leg	Yes	No
Left leg	Yes	No

3) In what part of the leg or buttock do you feel it?

a) Pain includes calf/calves

Right leg	Yes	No
Left leg	Yes	No

b) Pain includes thigh/thighs

Right leg	Yes	No
Left leg	Yes	No

c) Pain includes buttock/buttocks

Right leg	Yes	No
Left leg	Yes	No

4) Do you get it when you walk uphill or hurry?

Right leg	Yes	No
Left leg	Yes	No
Never walk uphill/hurry		

5) Do you get it when you walk at an ordinary pace on the level?

Right leg	Yes	No
Left leg	Yes	No

6) Does the pain ever disappear while you are walking?

Right leg	Yes	No
Left leg	Yes	No

7) What do you do if you get it when you are walking?

Right leg	Stop or slow down	Continue on
Left leg	Stop or slow down	Continue on

8) What happens to it if you stand still?

Right leg	Lessened or relieved	Unchanged
Left leg	Lessened or relieved	Unchanged

9) If lessened or relieved, how soon?

Right leg	10 min or less	More than 10 min
Left leg	10 min or less	More than 10 min

References

1. Marcoux RM, Larrat EP, Taubman AH et al. Screening for peripheral arterial disease. *J Am Pharm Assoc (Wash)* 1996;**NS36**:370–3.

2. Kannel W, Skinner JJ, Schwartz M et al. Intermittent claudication: incidence in the Framingham Study. *Circulation* 1970;**41**:875–83.

3. Leng GC, Lee AJ, Fowkes FG et al. Incidence, natural history and cardiovascular events in symptomatic and asymptomatic peripheral arterial disease in the general population. *Int J Epidemiol* 1996;**25**:1172–81.

4. Kornitzer M, Dramaix M, Sobolski J et al. Ankle/arm pressure index in asymptomatic middle-aged males: an independent predictor of ten-year coronary heart disease mortality. *Angiology* 1995;**46**:211–9.

5. Binaghi F, Fronteddu PF, Cannas F et al. Prevalence of peripheral arterial occlusive disease and associated risk factors in a sample of southern Sardinian population. *Int Angiol* 1994;**13**:233–45.

6. Stoffers HE, Rinkens PE, Kester AD et al. The prevalence of asymptomatic and unrecognized peripheral arterial occlusive disease. *Int J Epidemiol* 1996;**25**:282–90.

7. Criqui M, Fronek A, Barrett–Connor E et al. The prevalence of peripheral arterial disease in a defined population. *Circulation* 1985;**71**:510–5.

8. Newman A, Shemanski L, Manolio T et al. Ankle–arm index as a predictor of cardiovascular disease and mortality in the cardiovascular health study. *Arterioscler Thromb Vasc Biol* 1999;**19**:538–45.

9. Schroll M, Munck O. Estimation of peripheral atherosclerotic disease by ankle blood pressure measurements in a population study of 60–year-old men and women. *J Chron Dis* 1981;**34**:261–9.

10. Fowkes FG, Housley E, Cawood EH et al. Edinburgh Artery Study: prevalence of asymptomatic and symptomatic peripheral arterial disease in the general population. *Int J Epidemiol* 1991;**20**:384–92.

11. Sim EK, Koo G, Adebo OA et al. Prevalence of peripheral artery disease in patients with coronary artery disease. *Ann Acad Med Singapore* 1993;**22**:898–900.

12. Meijer WT, Hoes AW, Rutgers D et al. Peripheral arterial disease in the elderly: The Rotterdam Study. *Arterioscler Thromb Vasc Biol* 1998;**18**:185–92.

13. Newman A, Sutton–Tyrrell K, Vogt M et al. Morbidity and mortality in hypertensive adults with a low ankle/arm blood pressure index. *JAMA* 1993;**270**:487–9.

14. Curb JD, Masaki K, Rodriguez BL et al. Peripheral artery disease and cardiovascular risk factors in the elderly. The Honolulu Heart Program. *Arterioscler Thromb Vasc Biol* 1996;**16**:1495–500.

15. Bo M, Zanocchi M, Gallo R et al. Prevalence and risk factors of peripheral arterial disease among older patients living in nursing homes. *J Am Geriatr Soc* 1996;**44**:738–9 (letter).

16. Postiglione A, Cicerano U, Gallotta G et al. Prevalence of peripheral arterial disease and related risk factors in elderly institutionalized subjects. *Gerontology* 1992;**38**:330–7.

17. Fowkes FG, Housley E, Riemersma RA et al. Smoking, lipids, glucose intolerance, and blood pressure as risk factors for peripheral atherosclerosis compared with

ischemic heart disease in the Edinburgh Artery Study. *Am J Epidemiol* 1992;**135**:331–40.

18. Hiatt WR, Hoag S, Hamman RF. Effect of diagnostic criteria on the prevalence of peripheral arterial disease. The San Luis Valley Diabetes Study. *Circulation* 1995;**91**:1472–9.

19. Criqui M, Fronek A, Klauber M et al. The sensitivity, specificity, and predictive value of traditional clinical evaluation of peripheral arterial disease: results from non–invasive testing in a defined population. *Circulation* 1985;**71**:516–22.

20. Criqui MH, Denenberg JO, Bird CE et al. The correlation between symptoms and non–invasive test results in patients referred for peripheral arterial disease testing. *Vasc Med* 1996;**1**:65–71.

21. Criqui MH, Denenberg JO, Langer RD et al. The epidemiology of peripheral arterial disease: importance of identifying the population at risk. *Vasc Med* 1997;**2**:221–6.

22. Al Zahrani HA, Al Bar HM, Bahnassi A et al. The distribution of peripheral arterial disease in a defined population of elderly high–risk Saudi patients. *Int Angiol* 1997;**16**:123–8.

23. Dormandy J, Mahir M, Ascada G et al. Fate of the patient with chronic leg ischemia. *J Cardiovasc Surg*1989;**30**:50–7.

24. Valentine RJ, Grayburn PA, Eichhorn EJ et al. Coronary artery disease is highly prevalent among patients with premature peripheral vascular disease. *J Vasc Surg* 1994;**19**:668–74.

25. Mendelson G, Aronow WS, Ahn C. Prevalence of coronary artery disease, atherothrombotic brain infarction, and peripheral arterial disease: associated risk factors in older Hispanics in an academic hospital–based geriatrics practice. *J Am Geriatr Soc* 1998;**46**:481–3.

26. Alexandrova NA, Gibson WC, Norris JW et al. Carotid artery stenosis in peripheral vascular disease. *J Vasc Surg* 1996;**23**:645–9.

27. Cheng SW, Wu LL, Ting AC et al. Screening for asymptomatic carotid stenosis in patients with peripheral vascular disease: a prospective study and risk factor analysis. *Cardiovasc Surgery* 1999;**7**:303–9.

28. Cheng SW, Wu LL, Lau H et al. Prevalence of significant carotid stenosis in Chinese patients with peripheral and coronary artery disease. *Aust N Z J Surg* 1999;**69**:44–7.

29. Long TH, Criqui MH, Vasilevskis EE et al. The correlation between the severity of peripheral artery disease and carotid occlusive disease. *Vasc Medicine* 1999;**4**:135–42.

30. Jelnes R, Gaardsting O, Jensen K et al. Fate in intermittent claudication: outcome and risk factors. *BMJ* 1986;**293**:1137–40.

31. Leng GC, Fowkes FG, Lee AJ et al. Use of ankle brachial pressure index to predict cardiovascular events and death: a cohort study. *BMJ* 1996;**313**:1440–4.

32. Criqui MH, Langer RD, Fronek A et al. Mortality over a period of 10 years in patients with peripheral arterial disease. *N Engl J Med* 1992;**326**:381–6.

33. Criqui MH, Denenberg JO. The generalized nature of atherosclerosis: how peripheral arterial disease may predict adverse events from coronary artery disease. *Vasc Medicine* 1998;**3**: 241–5.

34. Caicoya Gomez–Moran M, Corrales Canel C, Lasheras Mayo C et al. [The association between a cerebrovascular accident and peripheral arterial disease: a case–control study in Asturias, Spain]. *Rev Clin Esp* 1995;**195**:830–5.

35. Tonelli C, Finzi G, Catamo A et al. Prevalence and prognostic value of peripheral arterial disease in stroke patients. *Int Angiol* 1993;**12**:342–3.

36. McKenna M, Wolfson S, Kuller L. The ratio of ankle and arm arterial pressure as an independent predictor of mortality. *Atherosclerosis* 1991;**87**:119–28.

37. Kannel W, McGee D. Update on some epidemiologic features of intermittent claudication. *J Am Geriatr Soc* 1985;**33**:13–8.

38. McDermott MM, Feinglass J, Slavensky R et al. The ankle–brachial index as a predictor of survival in patients with peripheral vascular disease. *J Gen Intern Med* 1994;**9**:445–9.

39. Pardaens J, Lesaffre E, Willems J et al. Multivariate survival analysis for the assessment of prognostic factors and risk categories after recovery from acute myocardial infarction: the Belgian situation. *Am J Epidemiol* 1985;**122**:805–19.

40. Pokorski RJ. Effect of peripheral vascular disease on long–term mortality after coronary artery bypass graft surgery. *J Insur Med* 1997;**29**:192–4.

41. Birkmeyer JD, O'Connor GT, Quinton HB et al. The effect of peripheral vascular disease on in–hospital mortality rates with coronary artery bypass surgery. Northern New England Cardiovascular Disease Study Group. *J Vasc Surg* 1995;**21**:445–52.

42. Birkmeyer JD, Quinton HB, O'Connor NJ et al. The effect of peripheral vascular disease on long–term mortality after coronary artery bypass surgery. Northern New England Cardiovascular Disease Study Group. *Arch Surg* 1996;**131**:316–21.

43. Criqui MH, Langer RD, Fronek A et al. Coronary disease and stroke in patients with large–vessel peripheral arterial disease. *Drugs* 1991;**42**(Suppl. 5):16–21.

44. Expert Panel on Detection Evaluation and Treatment of High Blood Cholesterol in Adults. Summary of the Second Report of the National Cholesterol Education Program (NCEP) Expert Panel on Detection, Evaluation, and Treatment of High Blood Cholesterol in Adults (Adult Treatment Panel II). *JAMA* 1993;**269**:3015–20.

45. Stein J, McBride P. Benefits of cholesterol screening and therapy for primary prevention of cardiovascular disease: A new paradigm. *J Am Board Fam Pract* 1998;**11**:72–6.

46. Eagle KA, Rihal CS, Foster ED et al. Long–term survival in patients with coronary artery disease: importance of peripheral vascular disease. The Coronary Artery Surgery Study (CASS) Investigators. *J Am Coll Cardiol* 1994;**23**:1091–5.

47. McDermott MM, Mehta S, Ahn H et al. Atherosclerotic risk factors are less intensively treated in patients with peripheral arterial disease than in patients with coronary artery disease. *J Gen Intern Med* 1997;**12**:204–15.

48. Avins AL, Browner WS. Improving the prediction of coronary heart disease to aid in the management of high cholesterol levels: What a difference a decade makes. *JAMA* 1998;**279**:445–9.

chapter two

Risk Factors

Joshua Beckman and Mark Creager

Introduction

The identification of atherosclerotic risk factors provides specific therapeutic targets for intervention to decrease the progression of peripheral arterial disease (PAD) and cardiovascular morbidity and mortality. Even in the absence of symptomatic peripheral arterial disease, risk factor modification is indicated to reduce cardiovascular morbidity and mortality.

Cigarette smoking

Among the traditional risk factors for atherosclerosis, cigarette smoking is most strongly correlated with the development of PAD. Several large studies have reported a 1.7–5.6 fold increased risk of developing PAD in smokers compared to non-smokers [1-6] (see Table 1). The impact of smoking on the prevalence of PAD varies according to the age of the population studied. In the Rotterdam Study, examining peripheral arterial disease in patients aged 55 years and older, 92% of the men and 45% of the women were current or former smokers [5]. In the Framingham Study, the incidence of intermittent claudication increased proportionally to the number of cigarettes smoked in both men and women [7]. Similarly, Bowlin and colleagues reported that the risk of intermittent claudication increased more than 2-fold over 5 years in patients who smoked more than 20 cigarettes per day compared to non-smokers [1]. The Reykjavik Study confirmed the importance of cigarette smoking. Not only did smoking increase the incidence of intermittent claudication by 8–10 fold, but a 32% decline in smoking in the population resulted in a 55% decrease in intermittent claudication [4]. The risk of amputation is also increased in

Table 1. Effects of cigarette smoking on PAD.					
First author	Country	Subjects	Age	Smoking group	Relative risk
Meijer [5]	The Netherlands	7715	>55	Current smokers	M 1.7 PAD
					F 1.2 PAD
Fowkes [6]	Scotland	1592	55–74	Current smokers	5.6 PAD
Kannell [7]	USA	5209	55–64	1–20 cigs	M 1.5 F 1.2 IC
				>20 cigs	M 3.9 F 1.8 IC
Bowlin [1]	Israel	8343	40–65	11–20 cigs	1.7 IC
				>20 cigs	2.2 IC
Smith [3]	UK	18,385	40–64	Current smokers	3.3 IC
Ingolffsson [4]	Iceland	3890	34–80	Current smokers	8–10 IC

cigs: Cigarettes Per Day; F: Female; IC: Intermittent Claudication; M: Male; PAD: Peripheral Arterial Disease.

smokers with PAD. In a Scandinavian vascular clinic, it was observed that patients with claudication who continued to smoke had a 16% risk of amputation over 7–10 years, while no amputations were required in those who stopped [8]. In another study of lower extremity bypass surgery, heavy smoking increased the risk of amputation 10-fold over moderate smoking [9]. In 124 claudicants studied over 10 months, smoking cessation alone increased ankle pressure by an average of 8.7 mmHg, and improved walking distance compared to those patients who continued smoking [10]. In patients with more severe disease who undergo catheter-based revascularization, smoking increases the rate of restenosis. Furthermore, rates of failure of surgical revascularization are increased among smokers. Among 160 patients who underwent femoral-popliteal bypass, 1-year patency rates for lower extremity bypass were 65% among smokers and 85% among non-smokers [11,12], and 5-year amputation rates were 28% versus 11% for smokers and non-smokers, respectively.

In addition to exacerbating the progression of PAD, cigarette smoking increases the likelihood of non-fatal and fatal cardiovascular events. In a

Table 2. Cigarette cessation rates after specific intervention.

Intervention	One year smoking cessation rate (%) *
None	0.1
Physician advice	2
Physician advice and extensive follow-up	5
Nicotine patch	16.4
Buproprion	30
Buproprion and nicotine patch	35.5

*Rates of cessation taken from references [14-18].

study of 343 consecutive claudicants who presented to a vascular clinic in Scandinavia, myocardial infarction (MI) occurred in 53% of the smokers and 11% of the non-smokers; 43% of the smokers had a cardiac death in contrast to 6% of the non-smokers [8]. In 133 patients who required surgical revascularization, Faulkner and colleagues reported a 3-year survival rate of 40% in patients who continued to smoke, compared to 67% in those who reported stopping [13]. In 190 patients who underwent revascularization, Lassilla et al. observed a 3-year survival rate of 40% for those who smoked more than 15 cigarettes per day and 65% for those who smoked less [9].

Smoking cessation is very difficult to achieve (see Table 2), because cigarette smoking is an addiction, akin to opiate dependence. Spontaneous cessation rates without intervention range from 2–5% in the USA [14], despite a desire to stop in nearly 75% of smokers [15]. Behavioral interventions can improve cessation rates, but not significantly. Five percent of patients who receive a physician's advice, follow-up correspondence, phone calls and supplementary visits will quit smoking in contrast to the 0.1% who do so without a physician's intervention [16]. Pharmacological interventions are more effective. There are two types of pharmacological therapies: nicotine replacement therapy and buproprion. Nicotine replacement may be obtained via a gum, patch, nasal spray or inhaler. In controlled studies, quit rates using these interventions vary between 17% and 48% at 6 months and 18% and 34% at 1 year [17]. Buproprion attenuates the desire for smoking via a poorly understood mechanism, and is associated with quit rates of 27–34.8 at 6 months and 23–30% at 1 year. In a trial of 732 smokers, which compared cessation rates when using buproprion, a nicotine patch, a placebo patch or both interventions, the quit rates at 1 year were 30.3, 16.4, 15.6 and 35.5%, respectively [18]. Buproprion therapy should be initiated 2 weeks prior to cigarette cessation and nicotine replacement should be started on the target quit date.

Diabetes mellitus

Epidemiological evidence has revealed that there is an association between diabetes mellitus and PAD (see Table 3). In the Rotterdam Study, diabetes was present in 11.9% and 16% of male and female patients with abnormal ankle-brachial indices (ABI), versus 6.7% and 6.3% for those without PAD [5]. The San Luis Valley Diabetes Study found evidence of at least single-vessel PAD in 12.1% of a population of Hispanic and Caucasian patients with type 2 diabetes mellitus [19]. In the Cardiovascular Health Study, diabetes was associated with a 3.8-fold increase in PAD patients aged over 65 [20]. In the Hoorn Study, prevalence rates were assessed in patients with normal glucose tolerance, impaired glucose tolerance, diabetes mellitus and diabetes mellitus requiring multiple medications [21]. A stepwise increase in the prevalence of PAD occurred in these groups, increasing from 7% in the normal glucose tolerance patients to 20.9% in patients with diabetes mellitus requiring more than one medication. An increased number of adverse events has also been reported in patients with diabetes in other studies [22-24].

Diabetes also increases the frequency of symptomatic PAD. In the Framingham patients, the risk of developing intermittent claudication in men with glycosuria was 350% greater than in non-diabetics, while in women there was an 860% increase in risk [25]. Furthermore, the duration of the diabetes is also associated with development of intermittent claudication [26]. Among 8343 Israeli men, the 5-year

Table 3. Effect of diabetes mellitus on PAD.

First author	Number of subjects	Subject age	Study group	Relative risk
Hiatt [19]	1710	20–74	Diabetics	1.6–3.1 PAD
Newman [20]	5084	>65	Diabetics	3.8 PAD
Beks [21]	5209	50–74	Diabetics on medication	3 PAD
Meijer [5]	7715	>55	Diabetics	M 1.8 PAD F 2.5 PAD
Kannel [25]	5209	55–84	Subjects with glycosuria	M 3.5 IC F 8.6 IC
Bowlin [1]	8343	40–65	Diabetics	1.9 IC

IC: Intermittent Claudication; PAD: Peripheral Arterial Disease.

incidence of intermittent claudication rose from 41.2:1000 in men without diabetes, to 76.2:1000 in men with diabetes [1].

Although females are generally less susceptible to PAD, the effect of diabetes on PAD development is so large as to eliminate the benefit of female gender. In the Framingham study, over a 20 year follow-up, diabetes increased the risk of femoral artery bruits and non-palpable pulses in women by 50%, thus attaining levels similar to those observed in men [27]. The importance of diabetes in females with PAD has also been demonstrated in Chinese patients [28].

Fifty percent of diabetic patients with toe pressures of 40 mmHg or less will develop rest pain, non-healing ulceration or gangrene within 2 years of diagnosis. In contrast, non-diabetics with PAD develop these complications at half this rate [29]. However, the association of symptomatic PAD with diabetes has not been observed in all investigations [30,31]. In the Edinburgh Artery Study, abnormal ABIs were associated with diabetes, but the relatively small number of patients with claudication did not show such an association [32].

Diabetes adversely affects outcomes in both percutaneous and surgical revascularization. In 137 patients who underwent femoro-popliteal angioplasty for critical limb ischemia, the diabetics had an 11-fold increase in the need for amputation [33]. Both primary and secondary patency following percutaneous transluminal angioplasty (PTA) and stent placement are diminished by diabetes [11,12,34,35]. Diabetic patients who undergo surgical revascularization have poorer functional status and quality of life than non-diabetic patients [36]. Also, the risk of MI and death after vascular surgery is increased in diabetics [37,38].

To date, no prospective trials have been performed to assess whether improved glycemic control decreases the cardiovascular risk associated with PAD, increases the walking distance of patients with intermittent claudication or decreases the need for amputation in affected patients. A retrospective review of the Diabetes Control and Complications Trial in patients with type 1 diabetes mellitus demonstrated a 22% risk reduction in the development of PAD events in the group that received intensive insulin therapy [39]. When combined with the reduction in coronary vascular events, there was a trend toward improvement associated with tight glycemic control. Epidemiological studies also validate the benefits of tight glycemic control [40].

The prospective Belfast Diet Study in type 2 diabetic patients demonstrated an increasing risk of MI of 1.04 per mmol increase in fasting plasma glucose [41]. In the United Kingdom Prospective Diabetes Study (UKPDS), 2693 subjects with type 2 diabetes were followed for nearly 8 years to evaluate baseline risk factors for coronary artery disease. Patients in the highest tertile of glycosylated hemoglobin had a 1.5-fold greater risk of MI compared to patients in the lowest tertile [42]. As yet, no prospective trial has demonstrated the benefits of improved glycemic control on lower extremity arterial events. However, improved glycemic control is recommended in patients with PAD. It may decrease the rate of cardiovascular events and is of proven benefit in preventing microvascular complications [43].

Table 4. Effect of elevated total cholesterol on PAD.			
First author	Subjects	Subject age (years)	Relative risk of PAD per TC increase
Murabito [44]	5209	45–84	1.2/40 mg/dl for IC
Ingolffson [4]	3890	34–80	1.007/mg/dl for IC
Newman [20]	5084	>65	1.1/10 mg/dl for PAD
Fowkes [6]	1592	55–74	1.6/50 mg/dl for IC
Bowlin [1]	8343	40–65	1.35/50 mg/dl for IC

IC: Intermittent Claudication; PAD: Peripheral Arterial Disease; TC: Total Cholesterol.

Hyperlipidemia

Elevated total cholesterol increases the risk of PAD (see Table 4), albeit not to the same extent as cigarette smoking and diabetes mellitus. Increased total cholesterol has been demonstrated in patients with PAD in the Edinburgh Artery [6], Framingham [25] and San Luis Valley studies [19], but the increase in risk is small. In the Cardiovascular Health Study, each 10 mg/dl increase in total serum cholesterol increased the risk of PAD 1.1-fold [20]. In the Rotterdam Study, total cholesterol was significantly elevated only among women with PAD [5]. Also, the subjects in the Speedwell [2] and Whitehall [3] studies who ultimately developed claudication tended to have higher cholesterol levels. The prospective evaluations of asymptomatic populations in Framingham [44], Iceland [4] and Israel [1] demonstrated a modestly increased risk of claudication associated with increased total cholesterol.

Components of the lipid profile, including low density lipoproteins (LDL), high density lipoproteins (HDL) and triglycerides, have been investigated to determine their role in PAD. The prevalence of PAD is increased in patients with familial hypercholesterolemia as compared to matched control subjects; in one study, 31% of patients with familial hypercholesterolemia had PAD, versus 3.7% of the control subjects [45]. Levels of LDL are higher in patients with PAD than in matched controls, and patients with PAD tend to have more atherogenic LDL [46,47]. The LDL tend to be smaller and denser, and are oxidized with elevated levels of plasma lipid peroxide. Oxidized LDL may play an important role in premature PAD [48].

Decreased levels of HDL are also associated with the development of PAD. Men with an abnormal ABI tend to have lower HDL levels [5], and those with a higher total cholesterol/HDL ratio are more likely to develop intermittent claudication [1]. In addition, patients with intermittent claudication have significantly lower median HDL cholesterol levels than matched controls [49,50]. Diminished HDL is also associated with a greater extent of atherosclerosis in the lower extremities [51].

The largest study conducted to investigate the relationship between triglycerides and PAD did not find any significant correlation with PAD or intermittent claudication on multivariate analysis [6]. Hypertriglyceridemia has been shown to be more common in patients with PAD than healthy controls [52,53], although not all reports are in agreement [49, 54]. In a vascular laboratory investigation, the patients with PAD were twice as likely to have hypertriglyceridemia [55]. This abnormality seems to occur more frequently in younger patients [56] and may be related to disease progression [57].

Therapy for dyslipidemias slows the progression of lower extremity atherosclerosis and decreases the onset of symptomatic disease. In one angiographic study, administration of cholestyramine, nicotinic acid or clofibrate (prescribed to lower lipid levels) induced a smaller increase in plaque size, progression and edge irregularity in the femoral artery [58]. However, the results of cholesterol lowering on angiographic endpoints have been mixed [59]. In the Program on Surgical Control of Hyperlipidemia, patients were randomized to partial ileal bypass to decrease their cholesterol by decreasing bile re-uptake. After 10 years, there was a statistically significant decrease in the number of patients with new intermittent claudication [60]. The Scandinavian Simvastatin Survival Study (4S) trial demonstrated the benefit of simvastatin on mortality and secondary prevention of MI in patients with an average cholesterol level of 260 mg/dl. A retrospective analysis of the data revealed that patients taking simvastatin were also less likely to develop intermittent claudication [61].

There have been no prospective trials of lipid lowering therapy in patients with PAD. However, the Coronary Drug Project has demonstrated the benefits of cholesterol lowering in the prevention of coronary artery disease morbidity and mortality [62]. The benefit of LDL lowering in secondary prevention of cardiovascular events was demonstrated in patients with elevated LDL levels in the 4S trial [63] and patients with average LDL levels in the Cholesterol and Recurrent Events (CARE) trial [64]. The importance of cholesterol in future morbidity and mortality was also demonstrated in asymptomatic patients [65,66].

Hypertension

Whereas hypertension and its control are strongly related to stroke incidence, the relationship to PAD is more modest and the benefits of blood pressure control are not established [1,67]. Novo et al. examined two epidemiological cohorts: the Trabia Study (835 subjects) demonstrated an increased frequency of hypertension in patients with PAD while the Casteldaccia Study (723 subjects) did not [55]. The Reykjavik Study did not find a relationship between hypertension and intermittent claudication in men [4], while the Edinburgh Artery Study found a 1.1 relative risk of claudication with increased systolic blood pressure [6]. In a review of risk factors associated with intermittent claudication using data obtained from the Framingham Heart Study, severe hypertension was associated with intermittent claudication. Patients with intermittent claudication had an odds ratio of 2.2 of having severe hypertension compared to controls, whereas moderate hypertension was found as commonly in patients as controls [44].

The effects of improved control of blood pressure on PAD may vary. In the Reykjavik Study, the decrease in frequency of hypertension in the population was significantly related to the observed decrease in PAD [4]. Furthermore, in the USA, a decrease in the prevalence of hypertension between 1983/84 and 1991/92 was associated with a decreased rate of lower extremity arterial reconstruction and amputation [68]. The effects of lowering blood pressure on the ability to walk in patients with intermittent claudication are mixed [69-71]. Small studies have demonstrated that the angiotensin converting enzyme (ACE) inhibitor, captopril, maintains and may increase walking distance in patients with claudication. α-adrenergic blockers, β-adrenergic blockers and calcium channel blockers may adversely affect walking distance, particularly if there is a substantial decrease in systolic blood pressure [70,71].

Hypertension was an independent predictor of late MI and death in patients who underwent lower extremity reconstruction [38]. The clear benefit to cardiovascular and cerebrovascular morbidity and mortality mandates the use of therapy in patients with PAD. The Joint National Committee report recommends the use of diuretics and β-adrenergic blockers as first-line agents in the treatment of hypertension [72].

Hyperhomocyst(e)inemia

Homocysteine is a sulfur-containing amino acid integral to the methionine metabolic pathway [73], and elevated levels are associated with PAD (see Table 5). Elevated levels of homocysteine were first noted to be associated with PAD in 1985 when Boers and colleagues examined 25 patients under the age of 50 with peripheral arterial atherosclerosis in the absence of hyperlipidemia, hypertension and diabetes mellitus [74]. Seven patients were heterozygous for homocysteinuria and had homocysteine levels above normal after methionine loading. In the Rotterdam Study of patients aged 55–74, those with elevated homocysteine tended to have a lower ABI than the rest of the population [75]. Elevated homocysteine is more prevalent in both elderly [76] and younger patients with PAD [77]. The severity of hyperhomocysteinemia is also related to the likelihood of PAD. In one study of 631 patients, each 5 μmol/l increment in total homocysteine increased the risk of PAD by 44% [78].

Table 5. Effect of hyperhomocysteinemia on PAD.

First author	Subjects	Subject age (years)	Homocysteine cut point (µM/l)	Effect on PAD	Other endpoints
Bots [75]	519	55–74	>18.6	ABI 5% lower	3-fold RR for CVD
Hoogeveen [78]	631	50–75	>14	44% increase in PAD/5 (µM/l) increase in Hcy	39% increase in CVD/5 (µM/l) Hcy
Cheng [79]	100 with sx and 100 controls	40–80	28.8 in patients	3.7-fold increase in PAD with sx	Unknown
Taylor [81]	351 with CVD and PAD	40–80	>14	Unknown	2.9-fold RR for death at 3 years

ABI: Ankle-Brachial Index; CVD: Cardiovascular Disease; Hcy: Homocysteine; PAD: Peripheral Arterial Disease; RR: Relative Risk; sx: Symptoms.

The relationship between elevated homocysteine and symptomatic PAD has been reported by several groups [78-80]. In the Homocysteine and Progression of Atherosclerosis Study, plasma homocysteine levels were greater in patients with PAD than in controls [81]. In an epidemiological study of 15,253 middle-aged men, 78 subjects with intermittent claudication were found to have higher plasma homocysteine levels than the other patients; 23% of the claudicants had levels above the 95th percentile for controls [82]. In the European Concerted Action Project, men in the highest quintile for plasma homocysteine had a relative risk of 2.2 for vascular disease [83].

Increased levels of homocysteine may also adversely affect the outcome of revascularization [77]. Hyperhomocysteinemia is more common in patients with vein graft stenoses compared to controls without stenoses [84]; however, others have reported no adverse effect on surgical outcome [85].

Elevated homocysteine levels are also predictive of cardiovascular and all-cause mortality [81,86]. Kark and colleagues examined the relationship between homocysteine and mortality in 1788 patients [87]. The relative risk of death in the highest versus lowest quintile was 2.0. In patients with symptomatic atherosclerosis, the effect of homocysteine was even greater, causing a 3.1-fold relative risk of death [81]. Therapy with folic acid, cobalamin and pyridoxine decreases homocysteine levels [88,89], but it is not known whether such treatment affects cardiovascular outcome. Several therapeutic trials are pending [90].

Obesity

The association between obesity and lower extremity arterial atherosclerosis has not been easy to establish. In the Framingham cohort of 5,209 subjects, relative weight was only a weak risk factor for claudication [25]. In fact, the association for cardiovascular death is significant only in marked obesity [91]. Obesity was not identified as a risk factor for PAD or intermittent claudication in the Edinburgh Artery Study [6], Whitehall Study [3] or Lipid Research Clinics Study [30]. Further investigation has revealed that certain types of obesity may confer an increased risk. Vogt and colleagues showed that only upper body or central obesity was an independent correlate for PAD in 1601 healthy elderly women [92], while the Framingham Study demonstrated a strong association between central obesity and coronary artery disease but not PAD in men [93].

Obesity may augment the risk of PAD by increasing the prevalence of the previously established risk factors. In a study of 8688 men followed for 5 years, being overweight was the most significant predictor of the development of type 2 diabetes mellitus [94]. Increasing body mass index has also been associated with increasing age, total cholesterol, blood pressure and fibrinogen levels [95].

Weight reduction is advised in patients with PAD. Wyatt and colleagues evaluated the maximum time patients with intermittent claudication could walk, while carrying various weights. They demonstrated a linear relationship of walking distance to claudication and load carried [96]. It follows that any decrease in weight will decrease the work required for walking and will improve exercise capacity.

Platelets

Although not clearly a risk factor for PAD, platelet activation has been consistently observed in populations with atherosclerosis for more than 20 years [97]. Increased ability of platelets to aggregate and byproducts of activation occur in patients with atherosclerosis [98-100]. Platelet activation has also been demonstrated in risk factors for atherosclerosis (e.g. smoking and blood pressure) [101] and may increase the concomitant oxidant stress [102].

Despite the lack of a proven causal relationship between platelet activation and atherosclerosis, antiplatelet administration is among the cornerstones of therapy in this patient population. Three approved agents have demonstrated efficacy in the prevention of vascular events: aspirin, ticlopidine and clopidogrel. The Antiplatelet Trialists' Collaboration (ATC) performed a meta-analysis of 46 randomized trials of antiplatelet therapy versus control, and 14 randomized trials comparing one antiplatelet regimen with another [103]. Of 15 studies in patients with PAD reviewed by the ATC, one demonstrated a 64% decrease in the incidence of arterial occlusion, 11 showed a combined 38% reduction in bypass graft occlusion, and two demonstrated an average 47% reduction in PTA restenosis with antiplatelet compared to control therapy [103,104]. Furthermore, in patients with symptomatic coronary artery disease, there was a significant decrease in second MI and death among those treated with antiplatelet medications. The Physicians Health Study prospectively confirmed the benefits of aspirin on PAD. In 22,071 patients, those taking aspirin (325 mg) every other day were 46% less likely to require peripheral arterial surgery [105]. Although, there does not seem to be any difference in outcome when using low or high dose aspirin, lower doses are better tolerated by patients [106,107]. Despite these prevention benefits, aspirin does not confer symptomatic improvement — walking distance is not improved by aspirin [108].

In several studies, ticlopidine, a thienopyridine derivative, increased walking distance in patients with claudication [69]. Ticlopidine also prevents untoward outcomes. The Swedish Ticlopidine Multicentre Study (STIMS) randomized 687 claudicants to ticlopidine (250 mg) twice daily or placebo and demonstrated that ticlopidine decreased the frequency of surgery by 51% [109]. Ticlopidine also improves bypass graft patency. In 243 patients who underwent lower extremity surgical revascularization randomized to ticlopidine or matching placebo, ticlopidine decreased the frequency of graft closure by one-third [110]. Patients with claudication, and those requiring surgery, both enjoyed a mortality benefit of ticlopidine compared to those patients on placebo [110-112]. Another thienopyridine derivative, clopidogrel, has been compared to aspirin. In a study of more than 19,000 patients with cerebrovascular, coronary and peripheral arterial disease, clopidogrel decreased the rate of ischemic stroke, myocardial infarction or vascular death by 8.7% compared to aspirin [113]. The patients with PAD had a 23.8% risk reduction in events, the greatest benefit of all three groups.

Oxidant stress

Atherosclerosis causes increased production of oxygen-derived free radicals [114]. Although, the pathogenic role of the free radicals in atherogenesis remains unclear [115], it has been demonstrated that risk factors for atherosclerosis augment oxidant stress [116-118]. There is also evidence that oxidative stress may exacerbate the progression of atherosclerosis [119]. It is in this emerging understanding of the role of oxygen-derived free radicals that enthusiasm for antioxidant therapy has taken root. Several antioxidants have undergone testing, including vitamin C (ascorbate), vitamin E (α-tocopherol) and β-carotene. Vitamin C is the most potent, endogenous, water-soluble antioxidant. Diminished plasma levels have been demonstrated in patients with coronary artery disease [120] and patients with PAD [121]. Acute administration of vitamin C has been demonstrated to decrease arterial stiffness and platelet 'aggregability', and to improve endothelial function [122,123]. Vitamin C, as part of a multi-antioxidant tablet, has not been demonstrated to improve walking distance, but did decrease the frequency of cardiovascular events [124]. Despite impressive epidemiological evidence that vitamin C intake is associated with decreased cardiovascular morbidity and mortality [125], there are no large clinical trials to demonstrate its role in the primary or secondary prevention of atherosclerosis and its complications.

Epidemiological evidence supports the benefits of vitamin E and β-carotene in prevention of complications of atherosclerosis [126-128]. Unfortunately, there is evidence that vitamin E does not prevent the development or progression of intermittent claudication [129,130]. Although one study demonstrated a significant reduction in MI [131], larger, randomized, double-blind studies have demonstrated that supplemental vitamin E and β-carotene do not confer any benefit in the prevention of non-fatal MI and death [132-134].

Renin-angiotensin system

All the necessary components of the renin-angiotensin system (RAS) exist in the endothelium. The local production of these substances is important in cell function, growth and death [135]. Different genetic polymorphisms and abnormal activation of the RAS are now considered potential risk factors for cardiovascular disease [136].

The benefits of ACE inhibitors have been examined in small studies of patients with PAD. In hypertensive patients, those receiving captopril had improved ankle perfusion pressure and walking distance at 8 weeks [69,137]. In a 6-month cross over trial of 20 hypertensive patients with PAD randomized to atenolol, labetalol, pindolol, captopril and placebo, only captopril maintained walking distance [71]. This seems to be a class effect, as enalapril also seems to improve lower extremity blood flow in patients with claudication [138].

Recent evidence has suggested that ACE inhibitors may cause a marked reduction in cardiovascular morbidity and mortality in patients with vascular disease. The Heart Outcomes Prevention Evaluation (HOPE) Study investigators randomized 9297 high-risk, non-hypertensive patients who had evidence of vascular disease or diabetes, plus one other cardiovascular risk factor, to ramipril or placebo [139]. Treatment with ramipril reduced absolute mortality by 16%, death from a cardiovascular cause by 26%, MI by 20% and stroke by 32%. Thus, for patients with any form of vascular disease, ACE inhibitors are important therapy. In the patients with PAD, there was a 22% reduction in the composite endpoint of MI, stroke or death.

Summary

The identification and treatment of risk factors should be considered for all patients with PAD. Antiplatelet therapy and interventions to decrease cigarette smoking, improve dyslipidemias, lower blood pressure and improve glycemic control will decrease cardiovascular morbidity and mortality and potentially reduce the risk of disabling claudication and amputation. Treatment strategies to modify emerging risk factors, such as hyperhomocysteinemia and oxidative stress, await the outcome of clinical trials.

References

1. Bowlin SJ, Medalie JH, Flocke SA et al. Epidemiology of intermittent claudication in middle-aged men. Am J Epidemiol 1994;**140**(5):418–30.

2. Bainton D, Sweetnam P, Baker I et al. Peripheral vascular disease: consequence for survival and association with risk factors in the Speedwell prospective heart disease study [see comments]. Br Heart J 1994;**72**(2):128–32.

3. Smith GD, Shipley MJ, Rose G. Intermittent claudication, heart disease risk factors and mortality. The Whitehall Study [see comments]. Circulation 1990;**82**(6):192–531.

4. Ingolfsson IO, Sigurdsson G, Sigvaldason H et al. A marked decline in the prevalence and incidence of intermittent claudication in Icelandic men 1968–1986: a strong relationship to smoking and serum cholesterol — the Reykjavik Study. J Clin Epidemiol 1994;**47**(11):1237–43.

5. Meijer WT, Hoes AW, Rutgers D et al. Peripheral arterial disease in the elderly: the Rotterdam Study. Arterioscler Thromb Vasc Biol 1998;**18**(2):185–92.

6. Fowkes FG, Housley E, Riemersma RA et al. Smoking, lipids, glucose intolerance and blood pressure as risk factors for peripheral atherosclerosis compared with ischemic heart disease in the Edinburgh Artery Study. Am J Epidemiol 1992;**135**(4):331–40.

7. Kannel WB, Shurtleff D. The Framingham Study. cigarettes and the development of intermittent claudication. Geriatrics 1973;**28**(2):61–8.

8. Jonason T, Bergstrom R. Cessation of smoking in patients with intermittent claudication. Effects on the risk of peripheral vascular complications, myocardial infarction and mortality. Acta Med Scand 1987;**221**(3):253–60.

9. Lassila R, Lepantalo M. Cigarette smoking and the outcome after lower limb arterial surgery. Acta Chir Scand 1988;**154**(11-12):635–40.

10. Quick CR, Cotton LT. The measured effect of stopping smoking on intermittent claudication. Br J Surg 1982;**69**(Suppl):S24–6.

11. King RB, Myers KA, Scott DF et al. Femoropopliteal vein grafts for intermittent claudication. Br J Surg 1980;**67**(7):489–92.

12. King RB, Myers KA, Scott DF et al. Aorto-iliac reconstructions for intermittent claudication. Br J Surg 1982;**69**(3):169–72.

13. Faulkner KW, House AK, Castleden WM. The effect of cessation of smoking on the accumulative survival rates of patients with symptomatic peripheral vascular disease. *Med J Aust* 1983;**1**(5):217–9.

14. Anthony JC, Warner LA, Kessler RC. Comparative epidemiology of dependence on tobacco, alcohol, controlled substances and inhalants: basic findings from the comorbidity survey. *Exp Clin Psychopharmacol* 1994;**2**:244–68.

15. Healthy People 2000 Review. Washington, DC: US Department of Health and Human Services 1994.

16. Law M, Tang JL. An analysis of the effectiveness of interventions intended to help people stop smoking. *Arch Intern Med* 1995;**155**:1933–41.

17. Okuyemi KS, Ahluwalia JS, Harris KJ. Pharmacotherapy of smoking cessation. *Arch Fam Med* 2000;**9**(3):270–81.

18. Jorenby DE, Leischow SJ, Nides MA et al. A controlled trial of sustained-release buproprion, a nicotine patch or both for smoking cessation [see comments]. *N Engl J Med* 1999;**340**(9):685–91.

19. Hiatt WR, Hoag S, Hamman RF. Effect of diagnostic criteria on the prevalence of peripheral arterial disease. The San Luis Valley Diabetes Study. *Circulation* 1995;**91**(5):1472–9.

20. Newman AB, Siscovick DS, Manolio TA et al. Ankle-arm index as a marker of atherosclerosis in the Cardiovascular Health Study. Cardiovascular Heart Study (CHS) Collaborative Research Group. *Circulation* 1993;**88**(3):837–45.

21. Beks PJ, Mackaay AJ, de Neeling JN et al. Peripheral arterial disease in relation to glycaemic level in an elderly Caucasian population: the Hoorn study. *Diabetologia* 1995;**38**(1):86–96.

22. Chowdhury TA, Lasker SS. Elevated glycated haemoglobin in non-diabetic patients is associated with an increased mortality in myocardial infarction. *Postgrad Med J* 1998;**74**(874):480–1.

23. Yudkin JS, Oswald GA, McKeigue PM et al. The relationship of hospital admission and fatality from myocardial infarction to glycohaemoglobin levels. *Diabetologia* 1988;**31**(4):201–5.

24. Feskens EJ, Kromhout D. Glucose tolerance and the risk of cardiovascular disease: the Zutphen Study. *J Clin Epidemiol* 1992;**45**(11):1327–34.

25. Kannel WB, McGee DL. Update on some epidemiologic features of intermittent claudication: the Framingham Study. *J Am Geriatr Soc* 1985;**33**(1):13–8.

26. Katsilambros NL, Tsapogas PC, Arvanitis MP et al. Risk factors for lower extremity arterial disease in non-insulin-dependent diabetic persons. *Diabet Med* 1996;**13**(3):243–6.

27. Abbott RD, Brand FN, Kannel WB. Epidemiology of some peripheral arterial findings in diabetic men and women: experiences from the Framingham Study. *Am J Med* 1990;**88**(4):376–81.

28. Cheng SW, Ting AC, Lau H et al. Epidemiology of atherosclerotic peripheral arterial occlusive disease in Hong Kong. *World J Surg* 1999;**23**(2):202–6.

29. Bowers BL, Valentine RJ, Myers SI et al. The natural history of patients with claudication with toe pressures of 40 mmHg or less. *J Vasc Surg* 1993;**18**(3):506–11.

30. Criqui MH, Browner D, Fronek A et al. Peripheral arterial disease in large vessels is

epidemiologically distinct from small vessel disease. An analysis of risk factors. *Am J Epidemiol* 1989;**129**(6):1110–9.

31. Da Silva A, Widmer LK, Ziegler HW et al. The Basle longitudinal study: report on the relation of initial glucose level to baseline ECG abnormalities, peripheral artery disease and subsequent mortality. *J Chronic Dis* 1979;**32**(11–12):797–803.

32. Fowkes FG, Housley E, Cawood EH et al. Edinburgh Artery Study: prevalence of asymptomatic and symptomatic peripheral arterial disease in the general population. *Int J Epidemiol* 1991;**20**(2):384–92.

33. Jeans WD, Cole SE, Horrocks M et al. Angioplasty gives good results in critical lower limb ischaemia. A 5 year follow-up in patients with known ankle pressure and diabetic status having femoropopliteal dilations. *Br J Radiol* 1994;**67**(794):123–8.

34. Capek P, McLean GK, Berkowitz HD. Femoropopliteal angioplasty. Factors influencing long-term success. *Circulation* 1991;**83**(2 Suppl):I70–80.

35. Stokes KR, Strunk HM, Campbell DR et al. Five-year results of iliac and femoropopliteal angioplasty in diabetic patients. *Radiology* 1990;**174**(3 Pt 2):977–82.

36. Holtzman J, Caldwell M, Walvatne C et al. Long-term functional status and quality of life after lower extremity revascularization. *J Vasc Surg* 1999;**29**(3):395–402.

37. Bergan JJ, Wilson SE, Wolf G et al. Unexpected, late cardiovascular effects of surgery for peripheral artery disease. Veterans Affairs Cooperative Study 199 [see comments]. *Arch Surg* 1992;**127**(9):1119–23; discussion 23–4.

38. Dawson I, van Bockel JH, Brand R. Late nonfatal and fatal cardiac events after infrainguinal bypass for femoropopliteal occlusive disease during a 31 year period. *J Vasc Surg* 1993;**18**(2):249–60.

39. Anonymous. Effect of intensive diabetes management on macrovascular events and risk factors in the Diabetes Control and Complications Trial. *Am J Cardiol* 1995;**75**(14):894–903.

40. Orchard TJ, Strandness DE, Jr. Assessment of peripheral vascular disease in diabetes. Report and recommendations of an international workshop sponsored by the American Heart Association and the American Diabetes Association 18–20 September 1992, New Orleans, Louisiana. *Diabetes Care* 1993;**16**(8):1199–209.

41. Hadden DR, Patterson CC, Atkinson AB et al. Macrovascular disease and hyperglycaemia: 10-year survival analysis in type 2 diabetes mellitus: the Belfast Diet Study. *Diabet Med* 1997;**14**(8):663–72.

42. Turner RC, Millns H, Neil HA et al. Risk factors for coronary artery disease in non-insulin dependent diabetes mellitus: United Kingdom Prospective Diabetes Study (UKPDS: 23) [see comments]. *BMJ* 1998;**316**(7134):823–8.

43. The effect of intensive treatment of diabetes on the development and progression of long-term complications in insulin-dependent diabetes mellitus. The Diabetes Control and Complications Trial Research Group. *N Engl J Med* 1993;**329**(14):977–86.

44. Murabito JM, D'Agostino RB, Silbershatz H et al. Intermittent claudication. A risk profile from The Framingham Heart Study. *Circulation* 1997;**96**(1):44–9.

45. Kroon AA, Ajubi N, van Asten WN et al. The prevalence of peripheral vascular disease in familial hypercholesterolaemia. *J Intern Med* 1995;**238**(5):451–9.

46. O'Neal DN, Lewicki J, Ansari MZ et al. Lipid levels and peripheral vascular disease in diabetic and non-diabetic subjects. *Atherosclerosis* 1998;**136**(1):1–8.

47. Sanderson KJ, van Rij AM, Wade CR et al. Lipid peroxidation of circulating low density lipoproteins with age, smoking and in peripheral vascular disease [published erratum

appears in Atherosclerosis 1996 Apr 5;121(2):295]. *Atherosclerosis* 1995;**118**(1):45–51.

48. Harris LM, Armstrong D, Browne R et al. Premature peripheral vascular disease: clinical profile and abnormal lipid peroxidation. *Cardiovasc Surg* 1998;**6**(2):188–93.

49. Horby J, Grande P, Vestergaard A et al. High density lipoprotein cholesterol and arteriography in intermittent claudication. *Eur J Vasc Surg* 1989;**3**(4):333–7.

50. Bradby GV, Valente AJ, Walton KW. Serum high-density lipoproteins in peripheral vascular disease. *Lancet* 1978;**2**(8103):1271–4.

51. Drexel H, Steurer J, Muntwyler J et al. Predictors of the presence and extent of peripheral arterial occlusive disease. *Circulation* 1996;**94**(9 Suppl):II199–205.

52. Mowat BF, Skinner ER, Wilson HM et al. Alterations in plasma lipids, lipoproteins and high density lipoprotein subfractions in peripheral arterial disease. *Atherosclerosis* 1997;**131**(2):161–6.

53. Kiesewetter H, Jung F, Kotitschke G et al. Prevalence, risk factors and rheological profile of arterial vascular disease; first results of the Aachen study. *Folia Haematol Int Mag Klin Morphol Blutforsch* 1988;**115**(4):587–93.

54. Mendelson G, Aronow WS, Ahn C. Prevalence of coronary artery disease, atherothrombotic brain infarction and peripheral arterial disease: associated risk factors in older Hispanics in an academic hospital-based geriatrics practice. *J Am Geriatr Soc* 1998;**46**(4):481–3.

55. Novo S, Avellone G, Di Garbo V et al. Prevalence of risk factors in patients with peripheral arterial disease. A clinical and epidemiological evaluation. *Int Angiol* 1992;**11**(3):218–29.

56. Strano A, Novo S, Avellone G et al. Hypertension and other risk factors in peripheral arterial disease. *Clin Exp Hypertens* 1993;**15**(Suppl 1):71–89.

57. Smith I, Franks PJ, Greenhalgh RM et al. The influence of smoking cessation and hypertriglyceridaemia on the progression of peripheral arterial disease and the onset of critical ischaemia. *Eur J Vasc Endovasc Surg* 1996;**11**(4):402–8.

58. Duffield RG, Lewis B, Miller NE et al. Treatment of hyperlipidaemia retards progression of symptomatic femoral atherosclerosis. A randomised controlled trial. *Lancet* 1983;**2**(8351):639–42.

59. Salonen R, Nyyssonen K, Porkkala E et al. Kuopio Atherosclerosis Prevention Study (KAPS). A population-based primary preventive trial of the effect of LDL lowering on atherosclerotic progression in carotid and femoral arteries. *Circulation* 1995;**92**(7):1758–64.

60. Buchwald H, Varco RL, Matts JP et al. Effect of partial ileal bypass surgery on mortality and morbidity from coronary heart disease in patients with hypercholesterolemia. Report of the Program on the Surgical Control of the Hyperlipidemias (POSCH) [see comments]. *N Engl J Med* 1990;**323**(14):946–55.

61. Pedersen TR. Coronary artery disease: the Scandinavian Simvastatin Survival Study experience. *Am J Cardiol* 1998;**82**(10B):53T–6T.

62. Canner PL, Berge KG, Wenger NK et al. Fifteen year mortality in Coronary Drug Project patients: long-term benefit with niacin. *J Am Coll Cardiol* 1986;**8**(6):1245–55.

63. Randomised trial of cholesterol lowering in 4444 patients with coronary heart disease: the Scandinavian Simvastatin Survival Study (4S) [see comments]. *Lancet* 1994;**344**(8934):138359.

64. Sacks FM, Pfeffer MA, Moye LA et al. The effect of pravastatin on coronary events after

myocardial infarction in patients with average cholesterol levels. Cholesterol and Recurrent Events Trial investigators [see comments]. *N Engl J Med* 1996;**335**(14):1001–9.

65. Shepherd J, Cobbe SM, Ford I et al. Prevention of coronary heart disease with pravastatin in men with hypercholesterolemia. West of Scotland Coronary Prevention Study Group [see comments]. *N Engl J Med* 1995;**333**(20):1301–7.

66. Downs JR, Clearfield M, Weis S et al. Primary prevention of acute coronary events with lovastatin in men and women with average cholesterol levels: results of AFCAPS/TexCAPS. Air Force/Texas Coronary Atherosclerosis Prevention Study [see comments]. *JAMA* 1998;**279**(20):1615–22.

67. Hooi JD, Stoffers HE, Kester AD et al. Risk factors and cardiovascular diseases associated with asymptomatic peripheral arterial occlusive disease. The Limburg PAOD Study. Peripheral Arterial Occlusive Disease. *Scand J Prim Health Care* 1998;**16**(3):177–82.

68. Feinglass J, Brown JL, LoSasso A et al. Rates of lower-extremity amputation and arterial reconstruction in the United States, 1979 to 1996. *Am J Public Health* 1999;**89**(8):1222–7.

69. Novo S, Abrignani MG, Pavone G et al. Effects of captopril and ticlopidine, alone or in combination, in hypertensive patients with intermittent claudication. *Int Angiol* 1996;**15**(2):169–74.

70. Solomon SA, Ramsay LE, Yeo WW et al. β-blockade and intermittent claudication: placebo controlled trial of atenolol and nifedipine and their combination. *BMJ* 1991;**303**(6810):1100–4.

71. Roberts DH, Tsao Y, McLoughlin GA et al. Placebo-controlled comparison of captopril, atenolol, labetalol and pindolol in hypertension complicated by intermittent claudication. *Lancet* 1987;**2**(8560):650–3.

72. Sheps SG. Overview of JNC VI: new directions in the management of hypertension and cardiovascular risk. *Am J Hypertens* 1999;**12**(8 Pt 2):65S–72S.

73. Malinow MR, Bostom AG, Krauss RM. Homocyst(e)ine, diet, and cardiovascular diseases: a statement for healthcare professionals from the Nutrition Committee, American Heart Association. *Circulation* 1999;**99**(1):178–82.

74. Boers GH, Smals AG, Trijbels FJ et al. Heterozygosity for homocystinuria in premature peripheral and cerebral occlusive arterial disease [see comments]. *N Engl J Med* 1985;**313**(12):709–15.

75. Bots ML, Launer LJ, Lindemans J et al. Homocysteine, atherosclerosis and prevalent cardiovascular disease in the elderly: The Rotterdam Study. *J Intern Med* 1997;**242**(4):339–47.

76. Aronow WS, Ahn C. Association between plasma homocysteine and peripheral arterial disease in older persons. *Coron Artery Dis* 1998;**9**(1):49–50.

77. Currie IC, Wilson YG, Scott J et al. Homocysteine: an independent risk factor for the failure of vascular intervention. *Br J Surg* 1996;**83**(9):1238–41.

78. Hoogeveen EK, Kostense PJ, Beks PJ et al. Hyperhomocysteinemia is associated with an increased risk of cardiovascular disease, especially in non-insulin-dependent diabetes mellitus: a population-based study. *Arterioscler Thromb Vasc Biol* 1998;**18**(1):133–8.

79. Cheng SW, Ting AC, Wong J. Fasting total plasma homocysteine and atherosclerotic peripheral vascular disease. *Ann Vasc Surg* 1997;**11**(3):217–23.

80. Taylor LM, Jr., DeFrang RD, Harris EJ, Jr. et al. The association of elevated plasma homocyst(e)ine with progression of symptomatic peripheral arterial disease. *J Vasc Surg* 1991;**13**(1):128–36.

81. Taylor LM, Jr., Moneta GL, Sexton GJ et al. Prospective blinded study of the relationship between plasma homocysteine and progression of symptomatic peripheral arterial disease. J Vasc Surg 1999;**29**(1):8–19; discussion 19–21.

82. Molgaard J, Malinow MR, Lassvik C et al. Hyperhomocyst(e)inaemia: an independent risk factor for intermittent claudication. J Intern Med 1992;**231**(3):273–9.

83. Graham IM, Daly LE, Refsum HM et al. Plasma homocysteine as a risk factor for vascular disease. The European Concerted Action Project [see comments]. JAMA 1997;**277**(22):1775–81.

84. Irvine C, Wilson YG, Currie IC et al. Hyperhomocysteinaemia is a risk factor for vein graft stenosis. Eur J Vasc Endovasc Surg 1996;**12**(3):304–9.

85. Valentine RJ, Jackson MR, Modrall JG et al. The progressive nature of peripheral arterial disease in young adults: a prospective analysis of white men referred to a vascular surgery service. J Vasc Surg 1999;**30**(3):436–44.

86. Nygard O, Nordrehaug JE, Refsum H et al. Plasma homocysteine levels and mortality in patients with coronary artery disease [see comments]. N Engl J Med 1997;**337**(4):230–6.

87. Kark JD, Selhub J, Adler B et al. Nonfasting plasma total homocysteine level and mortality in middle-aged and elderly men and women in Jerusalem [see comments]. Ann Intern Med 1999;**131**(5):321–30.

88. Omenn GS, Beresford SA, Motulsky AG. Preventing coronary heart disease: B vitamins and homocysteine [editorial; comment]. Circulation 1998;**97**(5):421–4.

89. Stein JH, McBride PE. Hyperhomocysteinemia and atherosclerotic vascular disease: pathophysiology, screening and treatment. Arch Intern Med 1998;**158**(12):1301–6.

90. Clarke R, Collins R. Can dietary supplements with folic acid or vitamin B6 reduce cardiovascular risk? Design of clinical trials to test the homocysteine hypothesis of vascular disease. J Cardiovasc Risk 1998;**5**(4):249–55.

91. Noppa H, Bengtsson C, Wedel H et al. Obesity in relation to morbidity and mortality from cardiovascular disease. Am J Epidemiol 1980;**111**(6):682–92.

92. Vogt MT, Cauley JA, Kuller LH et al. Prevalence and correlates of lower extremity arterial disease in elderly women. Am J Epidemiol 1993;**137**(5):55–95

93. Higgins M, Kannel W, Garrison R et al. Hazards of obesity — the Framingham experience. Acta Med Scand Suppl 1988;**723**:23–36.

94. Medalie JH, Papier CM, Goldbourt U et al. Major factors in the development of diabetes mellitus in 10,000 men. Arch Intern Med 1975;**135**(6):811–7.

95. Binaghi F, Fronteddu PF, Cannas F et al. Prevalence of peripheral arterial occlusive disease and associated risk factors in a sample of southern Sardinian population. Int Angiol 1994;**13**(3):233–45.

96. Wyatt MG, Scott PM, Scott DJ et al. Effect of weight on claudication distance. Br J Surg 1991;**78**(11):1386–8.

97. Cohen I. Role of endothelial injury and platelets in atherogenesis. Artery 1979;**5**(3):237–45.

98. Bodzenta-Lukaszyk A, Krupinski K, Dabrowski S et al. Blood platelet function in patients with obliterative arteriosclerosis of the lower limbs. Folia Haematol Int Mag Klin Morphol Blutforsch 1988;**115**(4):479–82.

99. Musumeci V, Rosa S, Caruso A et al. Abnormal diurnal changes in in vivo platelet

activation in patients with atherosclerotic diseases. *Atherosclerosis* 1986;**60**(3):231–6.

100. Wu KK. Platelet activation mechanisms and markers in arterial thrombosis. *J Intern Med* 1996;**239**(1):17–34.

101. Rohde LE, Hennekens CH, Ridker PM. Survey of C-reactive protein and cardiovascular risk factors in apparently healthy men. *Am J Cardiol* 1999;**84**(9):1018–22.

102. Gorog P, Kovacs IB. Lipid peroxidation by activated platelets: a possible link between thrombosis and atherogenesis. *Atherosclerosis* 1995;**115**(1):121–8.

103. Collaborative overview of randomised trials of antiplatelet therapy — I: Prevention of death, myocardial infarction, and stroke by prolonged antiplatelet therapy in various categories of patients. Antiplatelet Trialists' Collaboration [see comments] [published erratum appears in *BMJ* 1994 Jun 11;308(6943):1540]. *BMJ* 1994;**308**(6921):81–106.

104. Collaborative overview of randomised trials of antiplatelet therapy — II: Maintenance of vascular graft or arterial patency by antiplatelet therapy. Antiplatelet Trialists' Collaboration [see comments]. *BMJ* 1994;**308**(6922):159–68.

105. Goldhaber SZ, Manson JE, Stampfer MJ et al. Low-dose aspirin and subsequent peripheral arterial surgery in the Physicians' Health Study. *Lancet* 1992;**340**(8812):143–5.

106. Ranke C, Creutzig A, Luska G et al. Controlled trial of high- versus low-dose aspirin treatment after percutaneous transluminal angioplasty in patients with peripheral vascular disease. *Clin Investig* 1994;**72**(9):673–80.

107. Minar E, Ahmadi A, Koppensteiner R et al. Comparison of effects of high-dose and low-dose aspirin on restenosis after femoropopliteal percutaneous transluminal angioplasty. *Circulation* 1995;**91**(8):2167–73.

108. Ciocon JO, Galindo-Ciocon D, Galindo DJ. A comparison between aspirin and pentoxifylline in relieving claudication due to peripheral vascular disease in the elderly. *Angiology* 1997;**48**(3):237–40.

109. Bergqvist D, Almgren B, Dickinson JP. Reduction of requirement for leg vascular surgery during long-term treatment of claudicant patients with ticlopidine: results from the Swedish Ticlopidine Multicentre Study (STIMS). *Eur J Vasc Endovasc Surg* 1995;**10**(1):69–76.

110. Becquemin JP. Effect of ticlopidine on the long-term patency of saphenous-vein bypass grafts in the legs. Etude de la Ticlopidine apres Pontage Femoro-Poplite and the Association Universitaire de Recherche en Chirurgie [see comments]. *N Engl J Med* 1997;**337**(24):1726–31.

111. Janzon L, Bergqvist D, Boberg J et al. Prevention of myocardial infarction and stroke in patients with intermittent claudication; effects of ticlopidine. Results from STIMS, the Swedish Ticlopidine Multicentre Study [published erratum appears in J Intern Med 1990 Dec;228(6):659]. *J Intern Med* 1990;**227**(5):301–8.

112. Verhaeghe R. Prophylactic antiplatelet therapy in peripheral arterial disease. *Drugs* 1991;**42**(Suppl 5):51–7.

113. A randomised, blinded, trial of clopidogrel versus aspirin in patients at risk of ischaemic events (CAPRIE). CAPRIE Steering Committee [see comments]. *Lancet* 1996;**348**(9038):1329–39.

114. White CR, Brock TA, Chang LY et al. Superoxide and peroxynitrite in atherosclerosis.

Proc Natl Acad Sci U S A 1994;**91**(3):1044–8.

115. Halliwell B. The role of oxygen radicals in human disease, with particular reference to the vascular system. *Haemostasis* 1993;**23**(Suppl 1):118–26.

116. Scheffler E, Wiest E, Woehrle J et al. Smoking influences the atherogenic potential of low-density lipoprotein. *Clin Investig* 1992;**70**(3-4):263–8.

117. Kunsch C, Medford RM. Oxidative stress as a regulator of gene expression in the vasculature. *Circ Res* 1999;**85**(8):753–66.

118. Bruckdorfer KR. Oxidized lipoproteins. Baillieres *Clin Endocrinol Metab* 1995;**9**(4):721–37.

119. Ruef J, Peter K, Nordt TK et al. Oxidative stress and atherosclerosis: its relationship to growth factors, thrombus formation and therapeutic approaches. *Thromb Haemost* 1999;**82**(Suppl 1):32–7.

120. Vita JA, Keaney JF, Jr., Raby KE et al. Low plasma ascorbic acid independently predicts the presence of an unstable coronary syndrome. *J Am Coll Cardiol* 1998;**31**(5):980–6.

121. MacRury SM, Muir M, Hume R. Seasonal and climatic variation in cholesterol and vitamin C: effect of vitamin C supplementation. *Scott Med J* 1992;**37**(2):49–52.

122. Wilkinson IB, Megson IL, MacCallum H et al. Oral vitamin C reduces arterial stiffness and platelet aggregation in humans. *J Cardiovasc Pharmacol* 1999;**34**(5):690–3.

123. Levine GN, Frei B, Koulouris SN et al. Ascorbic acid reverses endothelial vasomotor dysfunction in patients with coronary artery disease [see comments]. *Circulation* 1996;**93**(6):1107–13.

124. Leng GC, Lee AJ, Fowkes FG et al. Randomized controlled trial of antioxidants in intermittent claudication. *Vasc Med* 1997;**2**(4):279–85.

125. Enstrom JE, Kanim LE, Klein MA. Vitamin C intake and mortality among a sample of the United States population [see comments]. *Epidemiology* 1992;**3**(3):194–202.

126. Losonczy KG, Harris TB, Havlik RJ. Vitamin E and vitamin C supplement use and risk of all-cause and coronary heart disease mortality in older persons: the Established Populations for Epidemiologic Studies of the Elderly. *Am J Clin Nutr* 1996;**64**(2):190–6.

127. Pandey DK, Shekelle R, Selwyn BJ et al. Dietary vitamin C and b-carotene and risk of death in middle-aged men. The Western Electric Study. *Am J Epidemiol* 1995;**142**(12):1269–78.

128. Virtamo J, Rapola JM, Ripatti S et al. Effect of vitamin E and β-carotene on the incidence of primary nonfatal myocardial infarction and fatal coronary heart disease. *Arch Intern Med* 1998;**158**(6):668–75.

129. Tornwall M, Virtamo J, Haukka JK et al. Effect of α-tocopherol (vitamin E) and β-carotene supplementation on the incidence of intermittent claudication in male smokers [published erratum appears in Arterioscler Thromb Vasc Biol 1998 Jul;18(7):1197]. *Arterioscler Thromb Vasc Biol* 1997;**17**(12):3475–80.

130. Tornwall ME, Virtamo J, Haukka JK et al. The effect of α-tocopherol and β-carotene supplementation on symptoms and progression of intermittent claudication in a controlled trial. *Atherosclerosis* 1999;**147**(1):193–7.

131. Stephens NG, Parsons A, Schofield PM et al. Randomised controlled trial of vitamin E in patients with coronary disease: Cambridge Heart Antioxidant Study (CHAOS) [see comments]. *Lancet* 1996;**347**(9004):781–6.

132. Rapola JM, Virtamo J, Ripatti S et al. Randomised trial of α-tocopherol and β-carotene supplements on incidence of major coronary events in men with previous myocardial infraction [see comments]. *Lancet* 1997;**349**(9067):1715–20.

133. Dietary supplementation with n-3 polyunsaturated fatty acids and vitamin E after myocardial infarction: results of the GISSI-Prevenzione trial. Gruppo Italiano per lo Studio della Sopravvivenza nell'Infarto miocardico [see comments]. *Lancet* 1999;**354**(9177):447–55.

134. Yusuf S, Dagenais G, Pogue J et al. Vitamin E supplementation and cardiovascular events in high-risk patients. The Heart Outcomes Prevention Evaluation Study Investigators. *N Engl J Med* 2000;**342**(3):154–60.

135. Gibbons GH. Endothelial function as a determinant of vascular function and structure: a new therapeutic target. *Am J Cardiol* 1997;**79**(5A):358.

136. Oparil S, Oberman A. Nontraditional cardiovascular risk factors. *Am J Med Sci* 1999;**317**(3):193–207.

137. Libretti A, Catalano M. Captopril in the treatment of hypertension associated with claudication. *Postgrad Med J* 1986;**62**(Suppl 1):34–7.

138. Sonecha TN, Nicolaides AN, Kyprianou P et al. The effect of enalapril on leg muscle blood flow in patients with claudication. *Int Angiol* 1990;**9**(1):22–4.

139. Yusuf S, Sleight P, Pogue J et al. Effects of an angiotensin-converting-enzyme inhibitor, ramipril, on cardiovascular events in high-risk patients. The Heart Outcomes Prevention Evaluation Study Investigators [see comments] [published erratum appears in N Engl J Med 2000 Mar 9;342(10):748]. *N Engl J Med* 2000;**342**(3):145–53.

chapter three

Pathophysiology

William Hiatt

Introduction

Peripheral arterial disease (PAD) is associated with an increased risk of overall cardiovascular mortality, and substantial morbidity resulting from claudication. The initial disease process is the result of atherosclerosis in the arterial circulation of the lower extremities, due to similar pathogenic mechanisms as those that cause coronary and cerebral atherosclerosis. Arterial occlusive disease results in reduced blood flow. In patients with claudication this is manifest during exercise, particularly in the calf muscles; in patients with critical leg ischemia, blood flow is inadequate to meet the resting demands of the limb. Importantly, altered hemodynamics do not completely explain the pathophysiology of claudication. Work from several laboratories has demonstrated secondary changes in the skeletal muscles of patients with PAD that are consistent with motor nerve injury, loss of type II muscle fibers and the presence of an acquired metabolic myopathy. Key findings include an alteration in the expression of mitochondrial enzymes, accumulation of metabolic intermediates, altered regulation of mitochondrial respiration, increased oxidative stress and the presence of somatic mutations in the mitochondrial genome. Understanding the structural and metabolic changes in skeletal muscle associated with PAD is important in understanding the pathophysiology of claudication and in the development of novel therapeutic strategies.

Peripheral arterial disease is one of the major manifestations of systemic atherosclerosis. The age-adjusted prevalence of PAD is approximately 12% in the adult population, and the disease is highly associated with the common cardiovascular risk factors of cigarette smoking, diabetes, hyperlipidemia, hypertension and elevations in homocysteine levels [1,2]. In patients with PAD, the co-existence of other clinical manifestations of cardiovascular disease (CVD) ranges from 5% in younger women to approximately 50–60% in older men [3]. However, when studied angiographically, the majority of patients with PAD also have severe coronary artery disease [4]. Thus, there is considerable evidence that patients with PAD have approximately the same risk of CVD mortality as those who have already had a myocardial infarction or stroke [5]. These data support the concept that patients with PAD have systemic atherosclerosis. No matter what regional circulation is most affected, all patients with atherosclerosis share common risk factors and pathophysiologic mechanisms.

Approximately 30–40% of all patients with PAD have classic symptoms of intermittent claudication or critical limb ischemia. Claudication is derived from a Latin word meaning "to be lame" or "to have a limp"; patients often develop a limp in the affected limb with the onset of claudication pain. This symptom is caused by reversible muscle ischemia and characterized by cramping and aching in the affected muscle. The discomfort develops during exercise, steadily increases during the walking activity to a point where the patient has to stop and is quickly relieved by rest without change of position. While classic Rose claudication (defined by a questionnaire) is uncommon, all patients with PAD have reductions in ambulatory activity and daily functional capacity [6]. Even asymptomatic PAD patients have a marked reduction in quality of life [7]. Therefore, the major goals of treatment are to prevent progression of systemic atherosclerosis leading to fatal and non-fatal ischemic events, to relieve the symptoms of claudication and to enhance quality of life.

An understanding of the pathologic mechanisms that underlie the development and progression of atherosclerosis and ischemic symptoms is critical in the overall management of the patient with PAD.

Pathogenesis of peripheral atherosclerosis

Mechanisms of atherosclerosis

Role of endothelial dysfunction
Experimental models of hypertension, hypercholesterolemia, diabetes or smoking are characterized by common endothelial abnormalities. The primary mediator of endothelial injury is thought to be oxidant stress from generation of the superoxide anion (O_2^-) [8,9]. This disrupts the cell membrane, increases endothelial permeability and stimulates expression of adhesion molecules (e.g. vascular cell adhesion molecule [VCAM-1]) and chemokines (e.g. monocyte chemo-attractant peptide [MCP-1]), factors that participate in monocyte adhesion and infiltration [10,11]. Therefore, one of the mechanisms by which cardiovascular risk factors may initiate atherosclerosis is induction of intracellular oxidative stress leading to endothelial injury.

Role of monocytes and macrophages
Following the initial endothelial injury, cellular elements such as monocytes and macrophages migrate into the subendothelium, begin to accumulate lipid and develop the appearance of foam cells. These cells become the initial stages of the arterial fatty streak. The activated monocytes release mitogens and chemo-attractants that recruit additional macrophages, as well as vascular smooth muscle cells, into the lesion. In addition, they generate reactive oxygen species that increase oxidative stress within the vessel wall, and accelerate oxidation of low density lipoprotein (LDL) cholesterol, leading to the promotion of foam cells [10,11]. As the cells accumulate in the subendothelial space, they distort the overlying endothelium and, eventually, may even rupture through the endothelial surface [11]. Macrophages also contribute to the thrombotic nature of the vulnerable plaque. The macrophages in the lesion are a source of tissue factor, which can be found in the acellular core as well as in the vascular smooth muscle of the fibrous cap [12]. Macrophage content and expression of tissue factor correlate with rupture of the human atherosclerotic plaque [12,13].

In areas of endothelial ulceration, platelets adhere to the vessel wall, releasing epidermal growth factor, platelet-derived growth factor and other mitogens that contribute to smooth muscle migration and proliferation. These factors induce smooth muscle cells in the vessel wall to proliferate and migrate into the area of the lesion. The muscle cells undergo a change in phenotype to secretory vascular smooth muscle cells, which elaborate extracellular matrix and transform the lesion into a fibrous plaque. The lesion grows with recruitment of more cells, elaboration of extracellular matrix and accumulation of lipid until it is transformed from a fibrous plaque to a complex plaque.

A fibrous cap overlying a necrotic core is a characteristic feature of the complex plaque. The necrotic core is composed of cell debris and cholesterol, and contains a high concentration of the thrombogenic tissue factor secreted by macrophages. In later stage lesions, calcification may occur, which accounts for the extensive amount of calcified deposits seen in larger peripheral arteries, such as the aorta, in patients with advanced PAD.

Role of infection
The causative factors initiating inflammation of the fibrous cap are unknown. However, there is mounting circumstantial evidence that implicates infection in the progression of atherosclerosis [14]. Sero-epidemiologic and immunohistochemical studies have shown that infectious agents such as cytomegalovirus, herpes virus or *Chlamydia pneumoniae* are associated with atherosclerotic vascular disease and vascular events [15-17]. Infection localizing to the plaque may activate endothelial cells to express adhesion molecules, stimulate vascular cells to undergo proliferation and/or induce resident inflammatory cells to elaborate cytokines that promote further local inflammation [14].

Role of ischemic exercise
Animal models have shown that both ischemia and ischemia-reperfusion are associated with marked oxidative stress due to the production of free radicals [18,19]. Reperfusion of ischemic myocardium also activates

neutrophils and platelets which further impair endothelial function [20]. When exercising, patients with claudication develop muscle ischemia; this is relieved by a relative reperfusion of the muscle with cessation of exercise. In patients with claudication, markers of oxidant stress are clearly elevated after single or multiple bouts of exercise [21,22]; e.g. malondialdehyde concentration (a marker of free radical generation) is elevated in PAD, and increases further with exercise [21,23]. The increased oxidant stress after ischemic exercise is associated with an increase in neutrophil count, and evidence of neutrophil and platelet activation [24,25]. Patients with PAD also have an increase in von Willebrand factor, which is a marker of endothelial injury [24,26]. Taken together, repeated episodes of claudication may promote systemic atherosclerosis by activating neutrophils and platelets and damaging vascular endothelium. Strategies to reduce or modulate the oxidant stress may be important not only to prevent atherosclerotic disease progression, but also to protect skeletal muscle from oxidant injury.

The risk factors and mechanisms listed above can lead to the development of atherosclerotic occlusive lesions in the abdominal aorta and peripheral vessels. These lesions are initially asymptomatic, but, when blood flow is sufficiently compromised, symptoms of claudication develop in the lower extremities. With advanced occlusive disease, blood flow is diminished at rest, and the patient develops more severe symptoms of ischemic rest pain or ischemic ulceration.

Pathophysiology of claudication

Hemodynamics

The arterial occlusive disease process initiates the pathophysiology of claudication and critical leg ischemia, with the hemodynamic severity of the lesions of primary importance in determining the clinical state. The major factors that determine reductions in flow with arterial disease include the length and internal radius of the stenosis, and blood viscosity. These parameters have been classically described by the Poiseuille equation:

$$\text{Pressure drop across the stenosis} = \frac{Q \times 8L\eta}{\pi r^4}$$

$$L = \text{length of stenosis; } \eta = \text{viscosity; } Q = \text{flow}$$

$$r = \text{internal radius of the stenosis}$$

This equation predicts that the radius or cross-sectional area of the stenosis is the dominant factor in determining the drop of pressure and flow across a stenosis. In addition, inertial loss of energy occurs as blood flow traverses a stenosis, which in part is related to the morphology of the stenosis and blood viscosity [27].

In PAD, a common angiographic finding is multi-level disease, e.g. a patient with mild claudication may only have iliac disease, but a patient with moderately severe claudication may have occlusive disease in the iliac and femoral circulations. Patients with critical leg ischemia almost always have disease affecting multiple arterial segments such as the iliac, femoral and tibial vessels. Based on the Poiseuille equation, an increase in the length of an individual stenosis will have an impact on blood flow and pressure drop. The hemodynamic effect of two equivalent lesions in series is double that of a single lesion [28]. In addition, several individual non-critical stenoses may become hemodynamically significant when combined in series in the same limb [28,29].

The hemodynamic significance of an arterial stenosis is a function of not only the percent stenosis, but also the flow velocity across the lesion [30,31]. At rest, blood flow velocity in the femoral artery may be as low as 10–20 cm/second, resulting in a calf blood flow of 1–2 ml/100 ml/min [32]. At this flow velocity, a stenosis will not become hemodynamically significant until it is 90% occlusive. Above 90% stenosis, flow and pressure rapidly decrease with increasing obstruction. However, with exercise in the normal extremity, flow velocity may increase to 150 cm/second, resulting in a calf flow of 15 ml/100 ml/min [32]. At these higher flow velocities, a stenosis of 50% would be hemodynamically significant. The major determinant of flow velocity in a regional circulation is the peripheral resistance of the vascular bed supplied by the major conduit vessels. Exercise is a major stimulus for peripheral vasodilatation. Thus, in a patient with a single iliac stenosis, there may be no symptoms at rest and the pulse exam may be normal. When flow velocity increases with exercise, the iliac lesion becomes hemodynamically significant, resulting in claudication symptoms and loss of pedal pulses due to the drop in pressure distal to the stenosis.

These hemodynamic changes are also utilized in assessing the ankle-brachial index or ABI.

A Doppler ultrasonic probe is used to detect systolic blood pressure in the ankle and arm. Patients with PAD will not only have an abnormal ABI at rest, but also exhibit a drop in ABI after exercise because of a reduction in ankle pressure compared to resting values. This drop in ankle pressure reflects not only the inability to increase limb flow appropriately across a fixed obstruction, but also an increase in flow velocity, which worsens the hemodynamic significance of the lesion.

Skeletal muscle

Peripheral arterial disease is not simply a hemodynamic disorder and the severity of symptoms cannot be explained entirely by the reduction in lower extremity perfusion. For example, the ABI or calf blood flow in claudicants is not well correlated with their exercise performance on a treadmill or the severity of symptoms in the community setting [34,35]. Also revascularization of the limb does not completely normalize exercise performance, and interventions such as exercise rehabilitation (which do not alter hemodynamics) have established efficacy [36,37]. Additional factors distal to the arterial obstruction that may impair limb function include ischemic injury to muscle and nerve, and alterations in skeletal muscle metabolism.

Histologic and neurologic effects of PAD
Skeletal muscle is primarily composed of two different fiber types. Type I oxidative, slow twitch fibers have large numbers of

mitochondria and are used to sustain repetitive muscle contractions, under aerobic conditions, over long periods of time. In contrast, type II glycolytic, fast twitch fibers have fewer mitochondria but generate more force during contraction. These fibers are used to produce rapid muscle contractions but are easily fatigued. Type II fibers have two sub-types: the IIa fiber has intermediate oxidative and contractile properties, while the IIb fiber has the least oxidative capacity but the greatest capacity for force generation. As the exercise requirement changes from sustained aerobic activity to a need for maximal force generation over a short duration, there is a progressive recruitment from type I to type II fibers. Thus in healthy muscle, exercise demands not only increased blood flow, but also coordinated neural control of the recruitment of appropriate muscle fiber types to meet the specific exercise conditions.

Several studies have demonstrated skeletal muscle injury in patients with chronic arterial occlusive disease, characterized as a distal axonal denervation leading to loss of muscle fibers and mild atrophy of the affected muscle [38]. Patients with claudication have a selective loss of type II glycolytic muscle fibers in the gastrocnemius muscle of the affected legs [39]. These observations were extended in a recent study where changes in skeletal muscle myosin isoforms were evaluated in patients with claudication and critical leg ischemia [40]. Skeletal muscle myosin isoforms, in part, determine the different muscle fiber types described above. The authors observed that patients with claudication had an isoform pattern similar to control subjects. Patients with ischemic rest pain had a moderate increase in type I isoform, no change in the IIa, but a decrease in the IIb isoform. Patients with ischemic ulcers had an increase in the type I myosin isoform with a corresponding decrease in both type IIa and IIb isoforms.

Changes in skeletal muscle isoforms and their corresponding fiber types may be important in terms of understanding how skeletal muscle adapts to chronic ischemia. Previous studies have shown that a decrease in type II fibers is associated with reduced muscle strength and muscle atrophy in the affected leg. Furthermore, the muscle weakness was correlated with reduced treadmill performance [39].

These results may explain, in part, why the reduced exercise performance in a patient with claudication cannot be entirely explained by alterations in limb blood flow and pressure. Treatments such as exercise training may address some of these pathologic changes by improving muscle strength and function [37].

Mitochondrial DNA injury

As described above, oxidant stress may contribute not only to the development of atherosclerosis, but also to skeletal muscle injury. Skeletal muscle mitochondria are at particular risk for oxidant injury to proteins critical for oxidative metabolism [41]. Mitochondria contain their own DNA, which encodes some of the proteins necessary for the electron transport chain [42]. Mitochondrial DNA is susceptible to injury, particularly with ischemic diseases such as PAD [42-44]; e.g. patients with PAD have an increased frequency of a mitochondrial DNA 4977 bp deletion mutation compared to age-matched control subjects [45]. However, this mitochondrial abnormality is not unique to muscle of the affected limb and is not correlated with exercise performance. Mitochondrial DNA deletions are not likely to be a primary factor in the pathophysiology of claudication, but rather reflect the systemic injury that occurs with increased oxidant stress.

Mitochondrial metabolic abnormalities

Mitochondria are the cellular sites of oxidative energy production, and thus play a key role in muscle energetics. Muscle mitochondrial content and activity reflects the functional state of the individual, increasing with exercise training and decreasing with prolonged bed rest or inactivity [46,47]. In healthy subjects, mitochondrial content is positively correlated with peak oxygen uptake, indicating the importance of muscle oxidative capacity in exercise performance of the individual [48]. In PAD, the marked limitation in walking activity alone would be expected to result in a decrease in muscle mitochondrial enzyme content and activity. In contrast, several studies have shown an increased mitochondrial content in the muscle of patients with PAD [49-51]. This increased mitochondrial expression appears to be a direct consequence of, and is proportionate to, the severity of the occlusive disease as assessed by leg hemodynamics [49].

Alterations in skeletal muscle mitochondria in PAD appear to reflect the severity of the underlying occlusive disease process. An increased mitochondrial content might improve oxygen extraction under ischemic conditions, or could reflect a compensatory mechanism for any intrinsic abnormality in mitochondrial oxidative capacity. However, mitochondrial content does not predict the functional capacity of the patient with claudication.

Accumulation of metabolic intermediates
Under normal metabolic conditions, fuel substrates such as fatty acids, proteins and carbohydrates are converted to acyl-coenzyme A (acyl-CoA) intermediates to be used in the Krebs cycle for complete oxidation. These coenzyme A-coupled intermediates are linked to the cellular carnitine pool through reversible transfer of acyl groups between carnitine and coenzyme A [52]. One of the functions of carnitine is to serve as a buffer to the acyl-CoA pool by formation of acylcarnitines. Therefore, during conditions of metabolic stress, incomplete oxidation or utilization of an acyl-CoA will lead to its accumulation. Transfer of the acyl group to carnitine will result in the accumulation of the corresponding acylcarnitine, which is easily measured [53].

In PAD, oxidative metabolism is severely impaired due to limited oxygen availability and mitochondrial injury. Subjects with unilateral claudication also have incomplete oxidation of fuel substrates, as evidenced by accumulation of acylcarnitines in the affected skeletal muscle [54]. Importantly, the unaffected leg in patients with unilateral claudication does not demonstrate acylcarnitine accumulation, demonstrating that this metabolic abnormality is specific to the limb with reduced blood flow. This accumulation of acylcarnitines implies that acyl-CoAs are not being efficiently oxidized, as the acyl-CoA pool and the acylcarnitine pool are in equilibrium. Acylcarnitine accumulation has functional significance, in that patients with the greatest accumulation had the lowest treadmill exercise performance [54]. Thus, the degree of metabolic abnormality (as defined by acylcarnitine accumulation) was a better predictor of treadmill exercise performance than the ABI, emphasizing the importance of altered skeletal muscle metabolism in the pathophysiology of claudication.

Altered control of mitochondrial respiration in PAD
A number of investigators have utilized ^{31}P magnetic resonance spectroscopy (MRS) to evaluate control of respiration in the muscle of control subjects and patients with PAD [55]. Using muscle ADP concentration as a marker of the state of mitochondrial respiration, mitochondrial function in PAD was characterized by an increased level of ADP to maintain cellular respiration. An increase in ADP concentration is unusual in human chronic diseases but is characteristic of classical mitochondrial myopathies [55]. These regulatory changes are consistent with the abnormal accumulation of oxidative intermediates and mitochondrial injury described in PAD.

References

1. Newman AB, Siscovick DS, Manolio TA et al., Cardiovascular Health Study Collaborative Research Group. Ankle-arm index as a marker of atherosclerosis in the cardiovascular health study. *Circulation* 1993;**88**:837–45.

2. Hiatt WR, Hoag S, Hamman RF. Effect of diagnostic criteria on the prevalence of peripheral arterial disease. The San Luis Valley Diabetes Study. *Circulation* 1995;**91**:1472–9.

3. Ness J, Aronow WS. Prevalence of coexistence of coronary artery disease, ischemic stroke, and peripheral arterial disease in older persons, mean age 80 years, in an academic hospital-based geriatrics practice. *J Am Geriatr Soc* 1999;**47**(10):125–56.

4. Hertzer NR, Beven EG, Young JR et al. Coronary artery disease in peripheral vascular patients. A classification of 1000 coronary angiograms and results of surgical management. *Ann Surg* 1984;**199**(2):223–33.

5. Newman AB, Shemanski L, Manolio TA et al. Ankle-arm index as a predictor of cardiovascular disease and mortality in the Cardiovascular Health Study. The Cardiovascular Health Study Group. *Arterioscler Thromb Vasc Biol* 1999;**19**(3):538–45.

6. McDermott MM, Mehta S, Liu K et al. Leg symptoms, the ankle-brachial index and walking ability in patients with peripheral arterial disease. *J Gen Intern Med* 1999;**14**(3):173–81.

7. Vogt MT, Cauley JA, Kuller LH et al. Functional status and mobility among elderly women with lower extremity arterial disease: the Study of Osteoporotic Fractures. *J Am Geriatr Soc* 1994;**42**(9):923–9.

8. Ohara Y, Peterson TE, Harrison DG. Hypercholesterolemia increases endothelial superoxide anion production. *J Clin Invest* 1993;**91**(6):2546–51.

9. Tsao PS, Buitrago R, Chang H et al. Effects of diabetes on monocyte-endothelial interactions and endothelial superoxide production in fructose-induced insulin-

resistant and hypertensive rats. *Circulation* 1995;**92**:A2666.

10. Berliner JA, Navab M, Fogelman AM et al. Atherosclerosis: basic mechanisms. Oxidation, inflammation, and genetics. *Circulation* 1995;**91**(9):2488–96.

11. Ross R. Cellular and molecular studies of atherosclerosis. *Atherosclerosis* 1997;**131**:S3–S4.

12. Moreno PR, Bernardi VH, Lopez-Cuellar J et al. Macrophages, smooth muscle cells and tissue factor in unstable angina. Implications for cell-mediated thrombogenicity in acute coronary syndromes. *Circulation* 1996;**94**(12):3090–7.

13. Little WC, Constantinescu M, Applegate RJ et al. Can coronary angiography predict the site of a subsequent myocardial infarction in patients with mild-to-moderate coronary artery disease? *Circulation* 1988;**78**(5 Pt 1):1157–66.

14. Libby P, Egan D, Skarlatos S. Roles of infectious agents in atherosclerosis and restenosis: an assessment of the evidence and need for future research. *Circulation* 1997;**96**(11):4095–103.

15. Grattan MT, Moreno-Cabral CE, Starnes VA et al. Cytomegalovirus infection is associated with cardiac allograft rejection and atherosclerosis. *JAMA* 1989;**261**(24):3561–6.

16. Saikku P, Leinonen M, Mattila K et al. Serological evidence of an association of a novel Chlamydia, TWAR, with chronic coronary heart disease and acute myocardial infarction. *Lancet* 1988;**2**(8618):983–6.

17. Minick CR, Fabricant CG, Fabricant J et al. Atheroarteriosclerosis induced by infection with a herpesvirus. *Am J Pathol* 1979;**96**(3):673–706.

18. Karmazyn M. Ischemic and reperfusion injury in the heart: cellular mechanisms and pharmacologic interventions. *Can J Physiol Pharmacol* 1991;**69**:719–30.

19. Turrens JF, Beconi M, Barilla J et al. Mitochondrial generation of oxygen radicals during reoxygenation of ischemic tissues. *Free Radic Res Commun* 1991;**12–13**(Pt 2):681–9.

20. Mehta JL, Nichols WW, Mehta P. Neutrophils as potential participants in acute myocardial ischemia: relevance to reperfusion. *J Am Coll Cardiol* 1988;**11**(6):1309–16.

21. Hickman P, Harrison DK, Hill A et al. Exercise in patients with intermittent claudication results in the generation of oxygen derived free radicals and endothelial damage. *Adv Exp Med Biol* 1994;**361**:565–70.

22. Ciuffetti G, Mercuri M, Mannarino E et al. Free radical production in peripheral vascular disease. A risk for critical ischaemia? *Int Angiol* 1991;**10**(2):81–7.

23. Belch JJ, Mackay IR, Hill A et al. Oxidative stress is present in atherosclerotic peripheral arterial disease and further increased by diabetes mellitus. *Int Angiol* 1995;**14**(4):385–8.

24. Edwards AT, Blann AD, Suarez-Mendez VJ et al. Systemic responses in patients with intermittent claudication after treadmill exercise. *Br J Surg* 1994;**81**(12):1738–41.

25. Kirkpatrick UJ, Mossa M, Blann AD et al. Repeated exercise induces release of soluble P-selectin in patients with intermittent claudication. *Thromb Haemost* 1997;**78**(5):1338–42.

26. Blann AD, Farrell A, Picton A et al. Relationship between endothelial cell markers and arterial stenosis in peripheral and carotid artery disease. *Thromb Res*

2000;**97**(4):209–16.

27. Young DF, Tsai FY. Flow characteristics in models of arterial stenoses. II. Unsteady flow. *J Biomech* 1973;**6**(5):547–59.

28. Flanigan DP, Tullis JP, Streeter VL et al. Multiple subcritical arterial stenoses: effect on poststenotic pressure and flow. *Ann Surg* 1977;**186**(5):663–8.

29. Karayannacos PE, Talukder N, Nerem RM et al. The role of multiple noncritical arterial stenoses in the pathogenesis of ischemia. *J Thorac Cardiovasc Surg* 1977;**73**(3):458–69.

30. Young DF, Cholvin NR, Kirkeeide RL et al. Hemodynamics of arterial stenoses at elevated flow rates. *Circ Res* 1977;**41**(1):99–107.

31. Demer L, Gould KL, Kirkeeide R. Assessing stenosis severity: coronary flow reserve, collateral function, quantitative coronary arteriography, positron imaging, and digital subtraction angiography. A review and analysis. *Prog Cardiovasc Dis* 1988;**30**(5):307–22.

32. Lewis P, Psaila JV, Morgan RH et al. Common femoral artery volume flow in peripheral vascular disease. *Br J Surg* 1990;**77**(2):183–7.

33. Carter SA. Clinical measurement of systolic pressures in limbs with arterial occlusive disease. *JAMA* 1969;**207**:1869–74.

34. Pernow B, Zetterquist S. Metabolic evaluation of the leg blood flow in claudicating patients with arterial obstructions at different levels. *Scand J Clin Lab Invest* 1968;**21**:277–87.

35. Hiatt WR, Nawaz D, Regensteiner JG et al. The evaluation of exercise performance in patients with peripheral vascular disease. *J Cardiopulmonary Rehabil* 1988;**12**:525–32.

36. Regensteiner JG, Hargarten ME, Rutherford RB et al. Functional benefits of peripheral vascular bypass surgery for patients with intermittent claudication. *Angiology* 1993;**44**:1–10.

37. Hiatt WR, Wolfel EE, Meier RH et al. Superiority of treadmill walking exercise vs. strength training for patients with peripheral arterial disease. Implications for the mechanism of the training response. *Circulation* 1994;**90**:1866–74.

38. England JD, Regensteiner JG, Ringel SP et al. Muscle denervation in peripheral arterial disease. *Neurology* 1992;**42**:994–9.

39. Regensteiner JG, Wolfel EE, Brass EP et al. Chronic changes in skeletal muscle histology and function in peripheral arterial disease. *Circulation* 1993;**87**:413–21.

40. Steinacker JM, Opitz-Gress A, Baur S et al. Expression of myosin heavy chain isoforms in skeletal muscle of patients with peripheral arterial occlusive disease. *J Vasc Surg* 2000;**31**(3):443–9.

41. Davies KJ, Delsignore ME. Protein damage and degradation by oxygen radicals. III. Modification of secondary and tertiary structure. *J Biol Chem* 1987;**262**(20):9908–13.

42. Wallace DC. Diseases of the mitochondrial DNA. *Annu Rev Biochem* 1992;**61**:1175–212.

43. Tritschler H-J, Meduri R. Mitochondrial DNA alterations as a source of human disorders. *Neurology* 1993;**43**:280–8.

44. Melov S, Shoffner JM, Kaufman A et al. Marked increase in the number and variety of

mitochondrial DNA rearrangements in aging human skeletal muscle. *Nucleic Acids Res* 1995;**23**(20):4122–26.

45. Bhat HK, Hiatt WR, Hoppel CL et al. Skeletal muscle mitochondrial DNA injury in patients with unilateral peripheral arterial disease. *Circulation* 1999;**99**(6):807–12.

46. Holloszy JO, Coyle EF. Adaptations of skeletal muscle to endurance exercise and their metabolic consequences. *J Appl Physiol* 1984;**56**:831–8.

47. Wibom R, Hultman E, Johansson M et al. Adaptation of mitochondrial ATP production in human skeletal muscle to endurance training and detraining. *J Appl Physiol* 1992;**73**(5):2004–10.

48. Wang H, Hiatt WR, Barstow TJ et al. Relationships between muscle mitochondrial DNA content, mitochondrial enzyme activity and oxidative capacity in man: alterations with disease. *Eur J Appl Physiol* 1999;**80**(1):22–7.

49. Jansson E, Johansson J, Sylven C et al. Calf muscle adaptation in intermittent claudication. Side-differences in muscle metabolic characteristics in patients with unilateral arterial disease. *Clin Physiol* 1988;**8**:17–29.

50. Lundgren F, Dahllof AG, Schersten T et al. Muscle enzyme adaptation in patients with peripheral arterial insufficiency: Spontaneous adaptation, effect of different treatments and consequences on walking performance. *Clin Sci* 1989;**77**:485–93.

51. Hiatt WR, Regensteiner JG, Wolfel EE et al. Effect of exercise training on skeletal muscle histology and metabolism in peripheral arterial disease. *J Appl Physiol* 1996;**81**:780–8.

52. Bieber LL. Carnitine. *Ann Rev Biochem* 1988;**57**:261–83.

53. Brass EP, Hoppel CL. Relationship between acid-soluble carnitine and coenzyme A pools in vivo. *Biochem J* 1980;**190**:495–504.

54. Hiatt WR, Wolfel EE, Regensteiner JG et al. Skeletal muscle carnitine metabolism in patients with unilateral peripheral arterial disease. *J Appl Physiol* 1992;**73**:346–53.

55. Kemp GJ, Taylor DJ, Thompson CH et al. Quantitative analysis by 31P magnetic resonance spectroscopy of abnormal mitochondrial oxidation in skeletal muscle during recovery from exercise. *NMR Biomed* 1993;**6**:302–10.

chapter four

Pharmacotherapy

Michael Jaff

Introduction

In the USA, from 1984–1999, the only pharmacologic therapy for PAD was pentoxifylline, which, although possessing data demonstrating superiority in improving initial and absolute claudicating distances, has offered minimal clinical benefit for patients.

However, as a result of impressive basic research into the pathophysiology of intermittent claudication, novel pharmacologic agents are being developed in order to improve walking distances and quality of life in patients with intermittent claudication.

Most physicians still recognize non-interventional therapy as the first option for patients without emergent need for revascularization. Unfortunately, non-interventional therapy has generally included only smoking cessation, control of hypertension, hypercholesterolemia and diabetes mellitus, and unsupervised exercise therapy — options that are only occasionally used by patients and methods that offer variable benefit. Historically, physicians have viewed these options as temporizing measures for patients who will ultimately endure revascularization or limb loss.

Non-interventional therapy for peripheral arterial occlusive disease is much more than unsupervised walking. Options for non-interventional therapy now include supervised exercise therapy, novel pharmacologic agents for intermittent claudication (IC) and angiogenic growth factors designed to improve limb salvage rates and walking distances (Figure 1). Aggressive risk factor modifications, such as tobacco cessation, normalization of hypercholesterolemia, control of hypertension and aggressive glycemic control in diabetes mellitus, are all important primary maneuvers in the care of patients with vascular disease, and should represent the cornerstone of treatment, even if revascularization is required [1] (see Chapter 2). Position papers reviewing the role of percutaneous revascularization for peripheral arterial occlusive disease support the initial role of risk factor modification and exercise [2].

Pharmacologic therapy for intermittent claudication

Drug therapy for lower extremity arterial occlusive disease, and specifically IC, has been viewed as ineffective. Between 1965 and 1985, 75 trials studied 33 pharmacologic agents to assess their efficacy as primary therapy for IC. Unfortunately, 75% of these trials were flawed by lack of a placebo-controlled arm, no double-blinding, inaccurate end points or small sample sizes [3].

Chelation therapy has generated many unsubstantiated claims of dramatic improvements in absolute claudicating distances. However, one double-blind, randomized, controlled trial of 32 patients with IC demonstrated no clinically significant increase in subjective and measured walking distances or ankle-brachial index (ABI) [4]. A thorough review of the published literature confirms the lack of scientific data supporting the use of a chelating agent as primary therapy for patients with IC [5].

Vasodilating agents

Vasodilator therapy has been disappointing as a treatment for patients with peripheral arterial occlusive disease. This is not surprising, given that the pathophysiology of PAD is not predominantly due to vasoconstriction, but rather to a complex series of interactions between flowing blood components, the endothelium and the subendothelial space. The overall benefit of vasodilator therapy has been weak. One recent short-term trial of

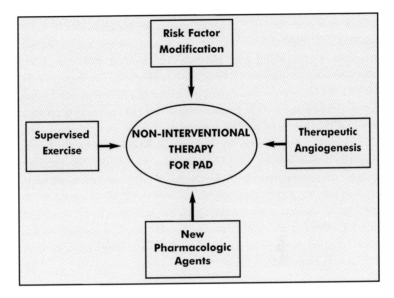

Figure 1. A comprehensive non-invasive approach to the management of patients with peripheral arterial disease and mild to moderate symptoms.

sublingual glyceryl trinitrate in patients with IC demonstrated a greater maximal walking distance, and a decrease in the fall of the ABI after exercise [6]. Verapamil has been shown to increase oxygen extraction in the ischemic limb. A short term, dose-ranging trial of slow-release verapamil in patients with moderate distance IC, revealed a 49% increase in maximal walking distance in those patients receiving verapamil as compared with placebo [7]. These and other vasodilator agents will require larger scale trials before their benefit for use in patients with PAD is widely accepted.

Antiplatelet agents

Antiplatelet therapy is an important adjunctive therapy for patients with PAD, predominantly as a method of preventing coronary and cerebrovascular events and death [8]. Ticlopidine and clopidogrel are thienopyridine derivatives that inhibit platelet aggregation. Ticlopidine has been shown to decrease the incidence of myocardial infarction

(MI), stroke and transient ischemic attacks in patients with IC [9]. In addition, as pharmacotherapy for IC, ticlopidine has demonstrated increases in the initial and absolute claudicating distances when compared to a placebo [10]. Finally, ticlopidine has been shown to improve the long-term patency of lower extremity saphenous vein bypass grafts. Patients assigned to placebo had a two year cumulative patency rate of 63%, compared to 82% in the ticlopidine-treated patients [11]. The Clopidogrel versus Aspirin in Patients at Risk for Ischemic Events (CAPRIE) trial evaluated 19,000 patients with a history of ischemic stroke, MI or symptomatic peripheral arterial occlusive disease, randomized to either clopidogrel or aspirin. Patients assigned to clopidogrel showed a statistically significant reduction in the combined primary endpoint of stroke, MI or vascular death compared to the aspirin-treated group. The greatest reduction was observed in patients with symptomatic PAD [12].

Prostaglandins

There has been considerable interest in prostaglandin E_1 (PGE_1) as a treatment for IC; studies comparing intravenous PGE_1 to exercise therapy or pentoxifylline have revealed significant benefits over comparable therapies. One outpatient study of 213 patients with IC, randomized to daily intravenous infusions of PGE_1 or placebo for two months, revealed an increase in treadmill walking distance of 101% with PGE_1 compared with 60% after placebo [13]. Studies with oral forms of PGE_1 are now in progress.

Metabolic agents

L-carnitine has biochemical effects that may offer significant advantages to patients with IC. Administration of L-carnitine in ischemic muscle causes an increase in total carnitine concentration in the muscle, as well as a decrease in plasma lactate levels. It appears that patients with severe IC have the highest concentrations of short-chain acylcarnitines in muscle and plasma. Higher total carnitine levels can deplete acetyl-CoA, which activates the acyl scavenger system and aids in removal of these acylcarnitines [14]. Recently, ex vivo studies of human fat arteries demonstrated that propionyl-L-carnitine (PLC) dilates arteries via prostaglandin-mediated, endothelium-dependent vasodilation [15].

PLC is effective in increasing walking capacity; in one double-blind dosing trial of 245 patients with IC, PLC caused a marked increase in walking capacity, and in the patients' view of quality of life, when compared with placebo [16]. A European study of 485 patients with claudication, stratified to severity of pain-free walking distance, revealed a marked improvement in initial and absolute claudicating distance. This reached statistical significance among patients with absolute claudicating distances <250 meters [17]. A large scale, North American trial is underway to study the benefits of this therapy further.

L-arginine has effects on synthesis of nitric oxide, which restores endothelium-induced vasodilation and is critical to blood pressure regulation and vascular tone. A recent study of 39 patients with IC, comparing intravenous infusions of L-arginine, PGE_1 or placebo, revealed a marked increase in pain-free walking distance by both active agents over the placebo. Normalization of endogenous nitric oxide formation was also seen but only with the L-arginine therapy [18]. Despite this, the clinical utility of L-arginine therapy remains unclear.

Hemorrheologic agents

Pentoxifylline was approved by the United States Food and Drug Administration for treatment of stable IC in 1984, and has remained the sole pharmacotherapy for patients in the USA until recently. Porter et al. evaluated 128 patients in a randomized, double-blind, placebo-controlled fashion and demonstrated a statistically significant increase in initial and absolute claudicating distances in patients assigned to pentoxifylline, compared to those receiving placebo [19]. Given the large number of clinical trials of varying scientific merit, a meta-analysis was performed to determine the true benefit of pentoxifylline in patients with IC [20]. The analysis suggests that pentoxifylline is effective in improving walking capacity of patients with moderate IC. However, when reviewing all trials, and all 'high-quality' trials, the results did not reach statistical significance.

Phosphodiesterase inhibitors

A significant advance in the pharmacologic therapy for patients with IC has been the advent of cilostazol, a chemically unique compound with several mechanisms of action. The most important of these are inhibition of platelet aggregation and vasodilation, via phosphodiesterase III inhibition. Cilostazol has been studied in over 12,000 patients worldwide, and clinical data have emerged demonstrating a marked improvement in walking distances over both placebo and pentoxifylline.

In one North American multicenter, randomized, double blind, placebo-controlled trial of 81 patients with chronic stable IC, 54 were assigned to cilostazol, and 27 received matching placebo. All patients were evaluated with a constant speed, constant grade treadmill test, and followed for 12 weeks. There was a 35% increase in initial claudicating distance (ICD), and a 41% increase in absolute claudicating distance (ACD) among patients who received cilostazol [21].

A dose-ranging trial compared doses of 50 or 100 mg cilostazol twice daily, versus placebo, in 394 patients with chronic stable IC. After 24 weeks, both doses of cilostazol demonstrated superiority in ACD and ICD when compared with placebo, with the 100 mg BID dose achieving optimal results [22].

In another randomized, prospective, double-blind trial of 239 patients with IC, 119 received 100 mg cilostazol orally, twice daily, and 120 received matching placebo. All patients were studied with constant speed, variable grade treadmill examinations, and followed on their assigned medications for 16 weeks. In addition, standardized quality of life indicators were assessed. Patients receiving cilostazol demonstrated a 96.4 meter increase in ACD, compared to only 31.4 meters in the placebo group [23].

Finally, a 24-week, multicenter, randomized, double-blind trial compared the effects of 100 mg cilostazol BID, 400 mg pentoxifylline TID and placebo in 698 patients with chronic stable claudication. Constant speed, variable grade treadmill testing was performed at 4-week intervals. Compared to placebo, cilostazol demonstrated a statistically significant increase in ICD (98.3 vs. 55.1%) and ACD (53.9 vs. 33.5%), whereas pentoxifylline did not (ICD 68.4 vs. 55.1%; ACD 30.4 vs. 33.5%). In addition, cilostazol was clearly and statistically significantly more effective in improving ICD and ACD than pentoxifylline [24]. As a result of these data, cilostazol has recently gained United States Food and Drug Administration approval for use in patients with chronic stable IC.

Angiogenesis/growth factors

Angiogenic growth factors have been isolated, identified and generated by recombinant gene technology in an effort to increase collateral arterial development in animal models of critical limb ischemia. This began with the intramuscular administration of recombinant fibroblast growth factor (FGF) and basic fibroblast growth factor (bFGF) to rabbits with acute hindlimb ischemia. After 14 days, there was marked augmentation of collateral vessel development compared to control limbs [25].

A similar animal model was used to investigate the role of vascular endothelial growth factor, VEGF, in improving collateral arterial development. Naked plasmid DNA, encoding VEGF, was applied to the hydrogel polymer coating of a balloon angioplasty catheter and the balloon was delivered percutaneously to the femoral artery. Not only did augmentation of collateral vessels occur, but improvement in calf blood pressure ratios was observed in those limbs treated with VEGF [26].

Direct intramuscular injection of naked plasmid DNA encoding VEGF was performed in the ischemic rabbit hindlimb model, and demonstrated dramatic augmentation in vascularity and improved perfusion to the ischemic limb [27]. As a result, human studies were performed, again utilizing naked plasmid DNA encoding VEGF, which was injected intramuscularly into ten limbs of nine patients with chronic critical limb ischemia and non-healing ulcers and/or ischemic rest pain. Although improved ABIs and augmentation in collateral vessel growth on contrast and magnetic resonance arteriography were found, the most impressive results were clinical. Ischemic ulcers either healed or markedly improved in four out of seven limbs, with limb salvage in three patients who were previously advised to undergo below-knee amputation [28].

Experimental models of bypass grafts have been performed in New Zealand White rabbits. Reversed jugular vein-to-common carotid artery vein grafts were submerged in solution containing VEGF or saline, implanted and then removed and histologically examined after 28 days. The vein grafts submerged in VEGF had a marked reduction in intimal thickness compared to saline treated grafts, suggesting that VEGF and other angiogenic growth factors may aid in graft patency [29]. A predictor of clinical efficacy of intramuscular VEGF therapy appears to be a patent dorsalis pedis artery, especially in patients with ischemic ulcerations [30].

Adjunctive percutaneous balloon angioplasty (PTA) and intra-arterial delivery of naked plasmid DNA encoding for VEGF has been performed in a small series of patients who underwent PTA of the superficial femoral artery. Of 19 patients in this cohort, VEGF was applied directly to the angioplasty site. After a mean follow-up of 9 months, 75% of angioplasty sites demonstrated no restenosis or minimal intimal hyperplasia [31].

A small series of patients with thromboangiitis obliterans (Buerger's disease) and ischemic ulcerations and/or ischemic rest pain received two intramuscular injections of phVEGF165 within 4 weeks. All five patients with digital gangrene demonstrated complete ulcer healing. One patient with rest pain had complete resolution. Two patients with extensive gangrene of the forefoot required below-knee amputation, despite having evidence by contrast and magnetic resonance arteriography of new collateral vessel growth [32].

Many planned controlled trials will provide further information on the clinical role and efficacy of angiogenesis, not only in patients with advanced peripheral arterial occlusive disease, but also in patients with lifestyle limiting disease.

Summary

Despite the enthusiasm for novel endovascular methods to revascularize patients with lower extremity arterial occlusive disease, the data documenting long-term improvement are somewhat limited. In addition, these procedures are accompanied by a small, but definite, risk of complications.

Risk factor modification (tobacco cessation, control of hypertension/hyperlipidemia/diabetes mellitus) must remain the cornerstone of therapy for PAD. However, supervised exercise rehabilitation, new pharmacologic agents (i.e. cilostazol) and modulation of angiogenesis could also assume primary therapeutic roles.

References

1. Weitz JI, Byrne J, Clagett GP et al. Diagnosis and treatment of chronic arterial insufficiency of the lower extremities: a critical review. *Circulation* 1996;**94**:3026–49.

2. Pentecost MJ, Criqui MH, Dorros G et al. Guidelines for peripheral percutaneous transluminal angioplasty of the abdominal aorta and lower extremity vessels. A statement for health professionals from a special writing group of the councils on cardiovascular radiology, clinical cardiology, and epidemiology and prevention, the American Heart Association. *Circulation* 1994;**89**:511–30.

3. Cameron HA, Waller PC, Ramsay LE. Drug treatment of intermittent claudication: a critical analysis of the methods and findings of published clinical trials, 1965-1985. *Br J Clin Pharmacol* 1988;**26**:569–76.

4. van Rij AM, Solomon C, Packer SGK et al. Chelation therapy for intermittent claudication. A double-blind, randomized, controlled trial. *Circulation* 1994;**90**:1194–9.

5. Ernst E. Chelation therapy for peripheral arterial occlusive disease. A systemic review. *Circulation* 1997;**96**:1031–3.

6. Walker SR, Tennant S, MacSweeney ST. A randomized, double-blind, placebo-controlled, crossover study to assess the immediate effect of sublingual glyceryl trinitrate on the ankle-brachial index, claudication, and maximum walking distance of patients with intermittent claudication. *J Vasc Surg* 1998;**28**:895–900.

7. Bagger JP, Helligsoe P, Randsback F et al. Effect of verapamil in intermittent claudication. A randomized, double-blind, placebo-controlled, cross-over study after individual dose-response assessment. *Circulation* 1997;**95**:411–4.

8. Antiplatelet trialists' collaboration. Collaborative overview of randomised trials of antiplatelet therapy-I: prevention of death, myocardial infarction, and stroke by prolonged antiplatelet therapy in various categories of patients. *Br Med J* 1994;**308**:81–106.

9. Janzon L, Bergqvist D, Boberg J et al. Prevention of myocardial infarction and stroke in patients with intermittent claudication;effects of ticlopidine. Results from STIMS, the Swedish Ticlopidine Multicentre Study. *J Intern Med* 1990;**227**:301–8.

10. Balsano F, Coccheri S, Libretti A et al. Ticlopidine in the treatment of intermittent claudication: a 21-month double-blind trial. *J Lab Clin Med* 1989;**114**:84–91.

11. Becquemin JP. Etude de la Ticlopidine apres pontage femoro-poplite and the Association Universitaire de recherche en Chirurgie. *N Engl J Med* 1997;**337**:1726–31.

12. CAPRIE steering committee. A randomised, blinded, trial of clopidogrel versus aspirin in patients at risk of ischaemic events (CAPRIE). *Lancet* 1996;**348**:1329–39.

13. Diehm C, Balzer K, Bisler H et al. Efficacy of a new prostaglandin E1 regimen in outpatients with severe intermittent claudication: results of a multicenter placebo-controlled double-blind trial. *J Vasc Surg* 1997;**25**:537–44.

14. Brevetti G, di Lisa F, Perna S et al. Carnitine-related alterations in patients with intermittent claudication. Indication for a focused carnitine therapy. *Circulation* 1996;**93**:1685–9.

15. Cipolla MJ, Nicoloff A, Rebello T et al. Propionyl-L-carnitine dilates human subcutaneous arteries through an endothelium-dependent mechanism. *J Vasc Surg* 1999;**29**:1097–1103.

16. Brevetti G, Perna S, Sabba C et al. Effect of propionyl-L-carnitine on quality of life in intermittent claudication. *Am J Cardiol* 1997;**79**:777–80.

17. Brevetti G, Diehm C, Lambert D et al. European multicenter study on propionyl-L-carnitine in intermittent claudication. *J Am Coll Cardiol* 1999; **34**:1618–24.

18. Boger RH, Bode-Boger SM, Thiele W et al. Restoring vascular nitric oxide formation by L-Arginine improves the symptoms of intermittent claudication in patients with peripheral arterial occlusive disease. *J Am Coll Cardiol* 1998;**32**:1336–44.

19. Porter JM, Baur GM. Pharmacologic treatment of intermittent claudication. *Surgery* 1982;**92**:966–71.

20. Hood SC, Moher D, Barber GG. Management of intermittent claudication with pentoxifylline: meta-analysis of randomized controlled trials. *Can Med Assoc J* 1996;**155**:1053–9.

21. Dawson DL, Cutler BS, Meissner MH et al. Cilostazol has beneficial effects in treatment of intermittent claudication. *Circulation* 1998;**98**:678–86.

22. Strandness DE, Dalman R, Panian S et al. Two doses of cilostazol versus placebo in the treatment of claudication: results of a randomized, multicenter trial. 71st Scientific Session, American Heart Association, Dallas, Texas, November, 1998 (Abstr.).

23. Money SR, Herd JA, Isaacsohn JL et al. Effect of cilostazol on walking distances in patients with intermittent claudication caused by peripheral vascular disease. *J Vasc Surg* 1998;**27**:267–75.

24. Dawson DL, Beebe HG, Davidson MH et al. Cilostazol or pentoxifylline for claudication? 71st Scientific Session, American Heart Association, Dallas, Texas, November, 1998 (Abstr.).

25. Baffour R, Berman J, Garb JL et al. Enhanced angiogenesis and growth of collaterals by in vivo administration of recombinant basic fibroblast growth factor in a rabbit model of acute lower limb ischemia: dose-response effect of basic fibroblast growth factor. *J Vasc Surg* 1992;**16**:181–91.

26. Isner JM, Walsh K, Symes J et al. Arterial gene therapy for therapeutic angiogenesis in patients with peripheral artery disease. *Circulation* 1995;**91**:2687–92.

27. Tsurami Y, Takeshita S, Chen D et al. Direct intramuscular gene transfer of naked DNA encoding vascular endothelial growth factor augments collateral development and tissue perfusion. *Circulation* 1996;**94**:3281–90.

28. Baumgartner I, Pieczek A, Manor O et al. Constitutive expression of phVEGF165 after intramuscular gene transfer promotes collateral vessel development in patients with critical limb ischemia. *Circulation* 1998;**97**:1114–23.

29. Luo Z, Asahara T, Tsurumi Y et al. Reduction of vein graft intimal hyperplasia and preservation of endothelium-dependent relaxation by topical vascular endothelial growth factor. *J Vasc Surg* 1998;**27**:167–73.

30. Isner JM, Blair R, Vale P et al. Patency of dorsalis pedis artery as a predictor of clinical outcome after intramuscular gene transfer of phVEGF165 in patients with non-healing ischemic ulcers. *71st Scientific Session, American Heart Association*, Dallas, Texas, November, 1998 (Abstr.).

31. Vale PR, Wuensch DI, Rauh GF et al. Arterial gene therapy for inhibiting restenosis in patients with claudication undergoing superficial femoral artery angioplasty. *71st Scientific Session, American Heart Association*, Dallas, Texas, November, 1998, (Abstr.).

32. Rauh G, Baumgartner I, Pieczek A et al. Treatment of Buerger's Disease by intramuscular gene transfer of phVEGF165. *71st Scientific Session, American Heart Association*, Dallas, Texas, November, 1998, (Abstr.).

chapter five

Surgery

Michael Lepore and Samuel Money

Introduction

Of the more than 1,000,000 patients who experience symptomatic disability secondary to atherosclerotic peripheral arterial disease (PAD) in the USA each year [1], a significant number may require surgical intervention. Conservative treatment can begin with simple modification of risk factors such as hyperlipidemia, hypertension and smoking. Institution of various exercise programs has also been shown to be beneficial, as evidenced by improved functional status and delayed surgical intervention [2]. As atherosclerotic disease may progress, a need for sound surgical evaluation and decision making may arise.

Patient evaluation

As with any diagnostic evaluation, a patient with PAD should provide a complete medical history and undergo a thorough physical examination. The planning of appropriate surgical treatment necessitates an understanding of the severity of disease. The physical exam will enable the astute clinician to identify the probable level, or levels, of atherosclerotic occlusive disease. Additional information can be provided by a good vascular laboratory, where the patient has been followed during attempts at conservative management of the PAD. The noninvasive vascular laboratory studies identify the affected arterial level of disease based upon segmental pressure changes at specified anatomic locations (high thigh, low thigh, calf, ankle) and the ankle-brachial index (ABI). The ABI is calculated by dividing the higher (posterior tibial or dorsalis pedis) Doppler-derived systolic pressure in each ankle by the higher of the two systolic Doppler-derived pressures in the arms. The number obtained correlates to the

Table 1. Assessment of methods used to evaluate functional status in persons with claudication.

Instrument	Strengths	Limitations	Recommendations
Ankle-brachial index (ABI)	Measure of disease severity In some studies, correlated with measures of functional status	Not strongly (or sometimes at all) correlated with measures of functional status in many studies	Use primarily to evaluate disease severity, only as a secondary marker of functional status
Treadmill test	Objective measure of walking ability Sensitive to treatment effect Reproducible	Relatively expensive Time/availability Does not measure community-based functional status	Use in clinical trials In clinical use only when objective endpoint is needed
Six-minute walk	Objective Somewhat reproducible Easily available Less expensive than treadmill	Limited validation data Not as reproducible as treadmill data Does not measure community-based functional status	Potentially useful as treadmill surrogate after more validation accomplished
Activity devices	Reflect daily ambulatory activity level	Limited validation data Subject to user capability	Use as research tool

From Regensteiner JG, Am J Med 1999 [3].

severity of disease. However, for patients experiencing claudication, the ABI (number) does not always directly correlate to symptomatology. Normal ABI is considered to be greater than 0.90, an index of 0.70–0.89 is indicative of some early atherosclerotic changes, 0.50–0.69 translates into more advanced disease, and an ABI less than 0.50 indicates advanced PAD. Once the ABI is in the 0.30–0.50 range or lower, there should be growing concern for critical limb ischemia progressing to gangrene and tissue loss. A high percentage of diabetics have medial calcinosis, thus limiting this noninvasive technique due to noncompressibility of the vessels.

Once the initial patient assessment is complete, noninvasive testing and the patient's current functional status must be taken into consideration (see Table 1) [3]. Peripheral circulation is more reliably assessed using a series of blood pressure cuffs and Doppler ultrasound, applied at different locations, at rest and post-exercise (see Figure 1). Post-exercise pressure decreases of greater than 20% have been shown to be indicative of hemodynamically significant stenoses [4]. Most, or all, of these tests are routinely performed in the noninvasive vascular laboratory. They have become an important part of monitoring not only the progression of arterial disease, but also the acute changes (i.e. decreases in ABI) that would factor in the decision to carry out early surgical intervention.

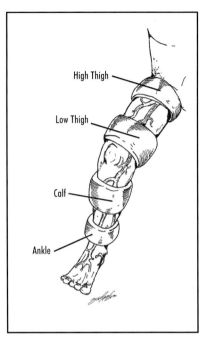

Figure 1. Segmental pressures.

Initially, a patient with intermittent claudication (IC) may be a good candidate for conservative treatment. Pharmacotherapeutic options continue to provide improved symptomatic relief and may eliminate surgical intervention for most patients. However, critical limb ischemia presenting as rest pain with or without tissue loss necessitates a more aggressive approach.

Arteriography provides a roadmap of occlusive disease. The revascularization may be through surgical bypass, percutaneous transluminal angioplasty (PTA) or percutaneous transluminal angioplasty with stent placement (PTAS).

There are three basic principles to follow:

1. arteriography should not be carried out unless either endovascular or surgical bypass is planned

71

2. arteriography must be complete from the infrarenal aorta to the pedal arches, with adequate visualization of runoff vessels

3. arterial disease is worse than it appears, because the angiogram is a two-dimensional view of a three-dimensional process [5]

Treatment

Vascular surgical guidelines recommend the treatment of proximal disease first, i.e. aortoiliac arterial occlusive disease, then femoropopliteal followed by tibioperoneal disease. Treatment of distal disease first will probably result in graft failure if adequate inflow is not present (e.g. femoropopliteal bypass while an ipsilateral significant iliac stenosis exists).

Aortoiliac disease

Anatomic patterns of occlusive disease in the aortoiliac region may be distinctly different from patient to patient. Three typical patterns have been described in the vascular literature [6]. Type I disease is localized aortoiliac disease with lesions confined to the distal aorta and common iliac vessels (Figure 2). In type II disease, the pattern of occlusive atherosclerosis is largely confined to the abdominal vessels, but also involves external iliac arteries and, perhaps, femoral arteries. Type III aortoiliac disease is the most common and is characterized by occlusive disease involving both aortoiliac inflow and infrainguinal outflow arterial segments.

There are a variety of options available for the treatment of aortoiliac occlusive disease, from percutaneous endovascular techniques to surgical bypass techniques. This has led to controversy regarding the optimum form of treatment. It is apparent that the outcome data of some competitive techniques, e.g. balloon angioplasty (with or without stent) versus aortobifemoral bypass, will continue to be explored. Most vascular surgeons adhere to some important principles when considering surgical intervention for aortoiliac occlusive disease:

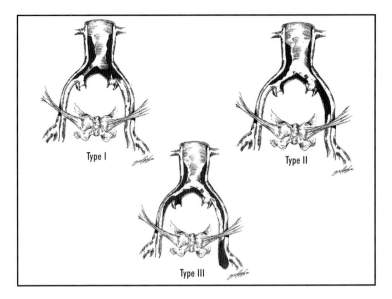

Figure 2. Patterns of aortoiliac disease.

1. aortic endarterectomy should be limited to younger patients with soft atheromatous plaques of the distal aorta and proximal iliac arteries. This procedure is extremely selective and not the most common form of treatment

2. the proximal anastomosis for aortobifemoral bypass should be based between the renal arteries and the inferior mesenteric artery

3. profundaplasty (patch angioplasty of the profunda femoris artery) is effective only if significant narrowing in an aortic reconstruction exists at the profunda origin, and if the profunda artery is patent

4. the need for concomitant distal bypass can usually be predicted preoperatively

5. axillofemoral bypass should be applied only in specific circumstances, although there are some surgeons who believe it can be applied more frequently [7-9]

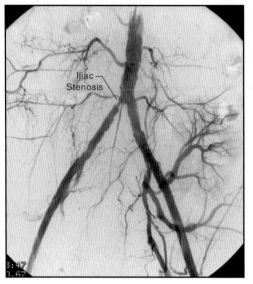

Figure 3. Angiogram demonstrating a short segment right-sided iliac stenosis.

Iliac Stenosis

Invasive treatment of aortoiliac disease may involve either endovascular or surgical techniques. Although the focus here is primarily on the surgical options, it is important to understand the basic anatomic differences that may make one patient more appropriate for surgical intervention versus endovascular interventions. PTA/PTAS is the preferred therapy for unilateral short segment (<5 cm) iliac stenosis or type I disease (see Figure 3). Success rates are reported to be 65–90% at 3–5 years and are considered somewhat comparable to those achieved by surgical aortofemoral reconstruction [10,11]. Overall, long-term patency rates of bypass grafts have been shown to be superior to those of stents, with hospital costs for the two techniques being similar. This has led some surgeons to believe that bypass is a more cost effective method of treatment [12]. On the other hand, there is little controversy regarding diffuse bilateral disease and/or long segment stenosis or occlusion (type II and III disease). These should be treated by aortobifemoral bypass, and not PTA/PTAS (see Figure 4). The greater majority of patients with aortoiliac disease fall into this category [6]. Since 1975, morbidity and mortality rates associated with aortobifemoral bypass have decreased to 8.0–12.4% and 1.0–3.0% aggregated risks, respectively, but

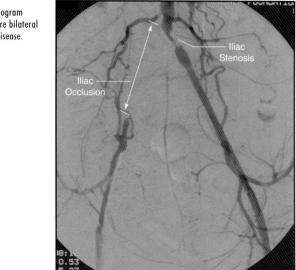

Figure 4. Angiogram depicting severe bilateral iliac arterial disease.

Iliac Stenosis

Iliac Occlusion

patency rates have remained fairly constant. Five-year patency rates of aortobifemoral bypass are reported to be 80–90% [13-15].

Patient selection for planned aortofemoral bypass is important due to the stress of the operation involving the need for aortic crossclamping. Infrainguinal disease should be carefully evaluated on the arteriogram to ascertain the necessity of a combined procedure (i.e. common femoral or profunda femoris disease). These patients are at increased risk for cardiac and cerebrovascular complications.

Once the decision has been made to proceed, the options regarding the type of graft should be considered. Dacron Y-aortic bifurcation grafts are the primary synthetic material used in this location. Various coatings have been applied (such as gelatin, collagen and albumin) but no statistically significant differences in intraoperative performance have been identified between these [16]. Polytetrafluoroethylene (PTFE) grafts are used for aortobifemoral bypass grafting by some surgeons. The largest prospective randomized study comparing dacron to PTFE revealed no statistical difference between the patency rates of the two materials. However, the investigators did report a higher rate of complications in the PTFE group and that a greater number of redo operations were required by this group [17]. It should be stressed that the choice of graft material is at the discretion of the respective surgeon.

Access to the aorta is gained through a midline abdominal incision, from xiphoid to pubis, with reflection of the small bowel. The duodenum is dissected free of the aorta and reflected cephalad and laterally. The proximal aortic anastomosis should be placed in a proximal, relatively disease-free segment of infrarenal aorta. The anastomosis can be performed as an end-to-end or end-to-side of graft to aorta. End-to-end anastomoses are performed in patients with aneurysmal disease or those with one patent external iliac artery. Once the aorta is divided, the distal aortic stump is oversewn (Figure 5A). The proximal anastomosis is then performed in a running fashion beginning on the back wall of the aorta (Figure 5B).

It is preferable to position the distal anastomoses at the level of the femoral arteries (Figure 5C). If the anastomosis is performed at the level of the external iliac artery, there is a higher risk of failure due to recurrent disease. The femoral arteries should be fully exposed through bilateral vertical groin incisions at the level of the inguinal ligament. Each limb of the graft is tunneled retroperitoneal and anterior to the iliac arteries down to the groin incisions. The common femoral, superficial femoral and profunda femoris arteries should be adequately exposed. Careful attention to, and correction of, any underlying profunda origin disease should be carried out at the time of the operation. The profunda femoris has been identified as a primary outflow vessel for aortobifemoral grafts by various authors. For this reason, it is of paramount importance for both early and late results that if any infrainguinal disease exists the graft hood is placed over the origin of the profunda [18-21].

Grafts placed in anatomical pathways that are different from those of native vessels are referred to as extra-anatomic bypass grafts. These are typically positioned to lower operative risk in patients with significant cardiac, pulmonary or cerebrovascular co-morbidities, or to avoid a hostile environment (e.g. infection, prior radiation or multiple abdominal operations). The two most commonly used extra-

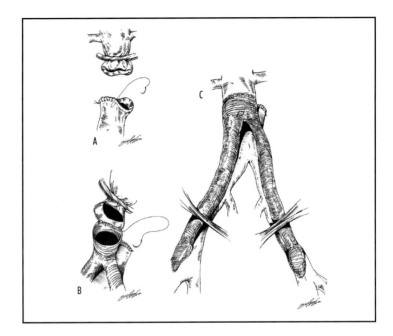

Figure 5. A. Diagram depicting the distal aortic stump being over-sewn. B. Running anastomosis beginning on the back wall of the aorta. C. Completed aortobifemoral bypass (end-to-end).

anatomic bypass grafts for aortoiliac occlusive disease are axillobifemoral and femorofemoral grafts [22].

The same bilateral femoral exposures are performed for the femorofemoral bypass graft placement. The operation is performed when unilateral occlusion (or stenosis) of an iliac artery occurs in the presence of a relatively disease-free contralateral iliofemoral vessel. Typically, a ringed (for reinforcement) graft is passed subcutaneously in the suprapubic region. Arterial inflow is provided by the iliac artery with outflow onto the contralateral common femoral/profunda femoris arteries (Figure 6) [23,24]. This operation is most frequently performed on patients who are at increased risk for an adverse event when undergoing any surgical procedure. The operative mortality has been reported to be between 0–8%, depending on the accompanying co-morbidities. Additionally, morbidity has been reported to range from 4–12% [25].

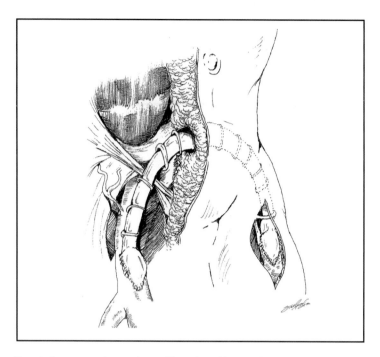

Figure 6. Representative diagram of a typical femorofemoral bypass graft.

Axillobifemoral grafts require the same bilateral groin exposure and are typically ringed PTFE grafts. The Y portion of the graft is tunneled subcutaneously in the same suprapubic location as the femorofemoral grafts. The straight portion of the graft is tunneled to the axillary artery, ipsilateral to the corresponding femoral artery with the most significant distal occlusive disease (see Figure 7). Morbidity and mortality rates have been reported to be 9.2 and 3.3%, respectively [15].

The patency rates of femorofemoral and axillobifemoral grafts are not as good as those of aortobifemoral bypass grafts, but they appear to be independent of synthetic graft material. Femorofemoral grafts have a reported 5 year patency rate of 65–75% [24]. Axillobifemoral 5-year patency results are reportedly worse, ranging from 50–55% [26, 27].

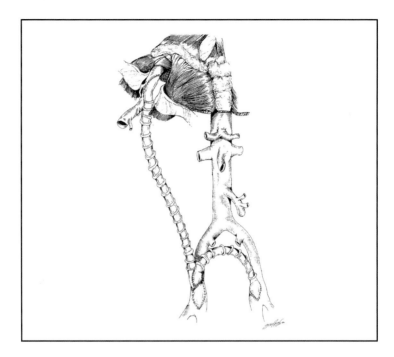

Figure 7. Completed axillobifemoral graft.

Infrainguinal disease

For reconstructive purposes, infrainguinal occlusive disease can be subdivided into three categories based on the position of the distal anastomosis: above-knee popliteal, below-knee popliteal and tibioperoneal arterial diseases. There is some disagreement regarding the net benefit of the use of a prosthetic for a first-time above-knee femoropopliteal bypass, in order to save the vein for a later, more distal bypass. The overall amputation-free survival has been shown to be superior if a vein is used as the bypass conduit at the initial operation. Additionally, a higher percentage of patients receiving a prosthetic first will require two operations [28]. If a vein is present it should be used as the first choice of conduit.

The most commonly used autogenous conduit for arterial bypass is the greater saphenous vein. It can be used in a reversed, non-reversed or *in situ* orientation. The specific vein orientation is again at the discretion of the respective vascular surgeon. There is some controversy over which method is superior and varying patency rates have been published. The differences in patency rates may be dictated by the selectivity and preferences of the reporting authors. Overall, patency rates are similar but the techniques remain different.

For either reversed (RSVG) or non-reversed saphenous vein grafts (NRSVG), the saphenous vein is harvested starting from the groin incision at the sapheno-femoral junction. The vein is gently dissected, taking care to situate the saphenectomy incision directly over the vein and avoid creating subcutaneous skin flaps that increase wound complications. The side branches are ligated and the appropriate saphenous vein length is harvested. At the completion of harvest, the vein is placed in saline. In the case of RSVG, the vein is then flushed under mild pressure and any defects are repaired with fine suture. For NRSVG, following proximal anastomosis, a valvulotome is used that ruptures all valves enabling prograde blood flow to occur in the conduit. Either conduit is then placed, or tunneled, into the respective location dictated by the arterial bypass [28,29].

The *in situ* technique is somewhat more involved, but is the most useful for distal bypass procedures. The two most common techniques are a semi-closed or an open technique. In the semi-closed technique, the greater saphenous vein is again identified at the sapheno-femoral junction during isolation of the femoral artery. The distal portion of the saphenous vein is also identified just proximal to the medial malleolus, attempting to incorporate the vein exposure into the distal bypass incision. Once the first couple of valves (near the sapheno-femoral junction) have been cut, the proximal femoral anastomosis is performed. The blood will then flow to the next competent valve and stop. A valvulotome is passed from the distal vein up to the most proximal valve and retracted distally to lyse the remaining valves. The distal vein is clamped gently. The side branches of the saphenous vein are identified by either on-table arteriography or ultrasonography in the semi-closed technique, or visually for the open technique. Small incisions are made directly over the side branches and the branches are ligated. Once all branches have been ligated, the distal anastomosis is performed. The open technique requires a full length incision but the rest of the principles are identical; lyse the valves, ligate side branches and perform the distal anastomosis [30].

The femoral to above-knee popliteal operation is performed for isolated superficial femoral artery occlusion or long segment stenosis in the presence of a relatively disease-free popliteal artery (see Figure 8). These patients typically present with claudication. They should only be offered operative intervention when risk factor modification, exercise programs and pharmacotherapy have failed to improve a significantly diminished lifestyle.

In femoral-popliteal bypass, exposure of the femoral artery is performed in the same way as has been described above. For the popliteal exposure, a medial longitudinal incision is made in the suprageniculate intermuscular groove just proximal to the medial femoral condyle. The fascia is incised to reflect the vastus medialis muscle anteriorly and the sartorius and adductors posteriorly. The space entered is the popliteal space as the superficial femoral artery exits Hunter's Canal and becomes the popliteal artery. The artery can be palpated lying just posterior to the femur and is isolated (see Figure 9) proximally and distally. The choice of synthetic graft material has not been shown to factor in overall patency [31]. The graft (whether synthetic or vein once prepared) is passed in the subsartorial plane from the popliteal space to the common femoral region. The graft is then sewn in following anticoagulation. Mortality rates are 0–1% with morbidity reported at approximately 6.5% including infectious, cardiac, pulmonary and neurologic complications.

It is generally accepted that synthetic graft should never be used below the knee unless no vein is available and the bypass is for limb salvage. The primary patency rates for femoral to distal bypass at 3 and 5 years have been shown to be 71 and 61%, respectively, for autogenous vein grafts, versus 12% for PTFE [32,33]. Mortality rates for this procedure are similar to above-knee bypass at 0–1%. Morbidity,

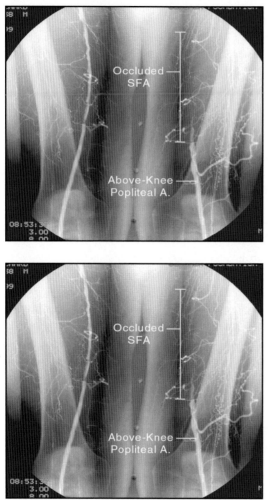

Figure 8. Angiogram demonstrating a left-sided SFA occlusion with reconstitution to the above-knee popliteal artery.

however, varies significantly between 6–30% depending upon the amount of preoperative ischemia, infection, or tissue necrosis present prior to bypass. A large study comparing reversed saphenous vein to in situ saphenous vein for distal bypass (below-knee) procedures revealed no statistically significant difference in primary patency rates [34].

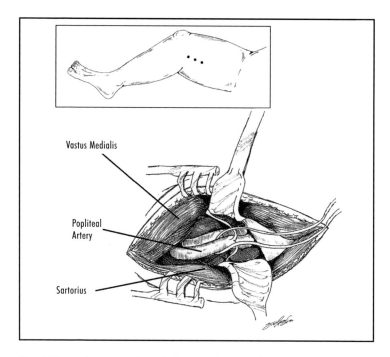

Vastus Medialis

Popliteal
Artery

Sartorius

Figure 9. Diagram demonstrating the standard incision with exposure of the above-knee popliteal artery.

Femoral to below-knee popliteal arterial bypass is typically indicated in patients with superficial femoral or popliteal artery occlusion, or hemodynamically significant stenoses reconstituting to the below-knee popliteal region (see Figure 10). The femoral artery is exposed and the saphenous vein harvested by the techniques described. The below-knee popliteal artery is exposed through a longitudinal medial calf incision posterior to the medial femoral condyle and extending distally to the tibial crest. An attempt should be made to orient the incision over the saphenous vein, so as to minimize undermining of the cutaneous flaps. The deep muscular fascia is incised subsequently reflecting the medial head of the gastrocnemius muscle posterolaterally to expose the popliteal fossa. The popliteal artery is then dissected free (Figure 11) from the tibial nerve and popliteal vein. Distal extension of the

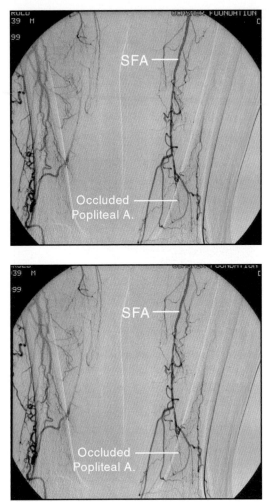

Figure 10. Angiogram demonstrating an occluded popliteal artery with collaterals to the below-knee popliteal artery.

incision along the anteromedial surface of the artery to transect the overlying musculotendinous origin of the semitendinosus, soleus and semimembranous muscles will expose the tibioperoneal trunk. Once the popliteal artery is exposed, the vein can be tunneled down the leg in a variety of ways. The two anastomoses are then performed.

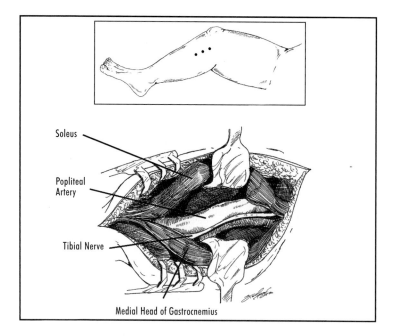

Soleus

Popliteal
Artery

Tibial Nerve

Medial Head of Gastrocnemius

Figure 11. Diagram that depicts the typical incision and exposure of the below-knee popliteal artery.

Distal exposure to the tibial and peroneal vessels is best obtained through individual incisions (see Figure 12). Isolation of the distal posterior tibial artery is achieved by a longitudinal incision on the medial aspect of the leg proximal to the medial malleolus. Approach to the anterior tibial artery requires a longitudinal incision over the anterior compartment in the distal third of the leg. The digital extensor and peroneal muscles are reflected laterally, while reflecting the anterior tibial muscle anteromedially to expose the vessel. The peroneal artery can be exposed through a longitudinal incision overlying the distal fibula. The flexor hallucis longus and peroneus longus muscles are reflected posteriorly after mobilization from the bone. A 5–10 cm segment of fibula is removed. Tedious dissection through the thin layer of fascia on the surface of the posterior tibial muscle will expose the peroneal artery [35]. Also, some surgeons prefer a medial approach to this vessel.

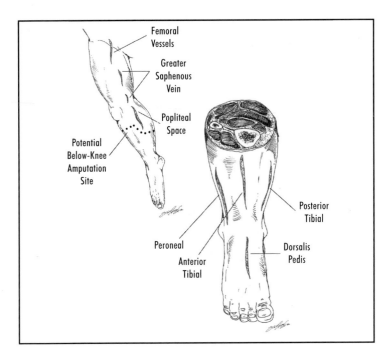

Figure 12. The most commonly used incisions for exposure of the distal lower extremity vessels.

Patients who require distal bypass to the above vascular location will have significant and possibly concurrent superficial femoral, popliteal and tibioperoneal arterial occlusive disease (see Figure 13). The orientation of the graft in the subcutaneous space (medial or lateral) will be dependent upon the respective vessel targeted for planned bypass. The surgical principles do not change. In addition, completion angiography is performed intraoperatively on nearly all distal bypass procedures.

It should be mentioned that profundaplasty is also an important tool for the patient with nonreconstructable disease, given the collateral circulation it can provide. Profundaplasty has long been reported as a first attempt alternative in patients with severe ischemia [36-38]. Additionally, it has been reported to provide vascular support to an amputation for healing purposes.

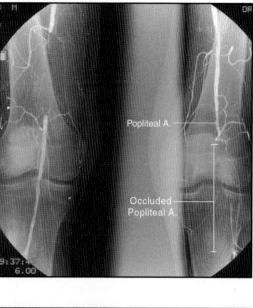

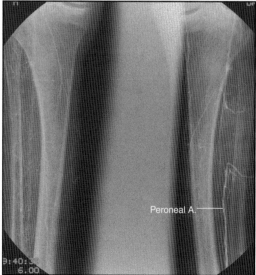

Figure 13. Angiogram demonstrating popliteal artery and
tibioperoneal occlusion with reconstitution to the peroneal artery.

Graft surveillance and graft salvage

Post-operatively, patients are monitored closely with vascular examination every 1–2 hours for the first 12 hours. Immediately post-operatively, the ABI is routinely performed and graft velocities are obtained after the patient has recovered further. The ultrasound probe is placed over the region of the graft and velocities are measured just proximal to the proximal anastomosis, in the mid-graft region and distal to the distal anastomosis, in an attempt to identify significant changes in velocities. When the graft has been recently placed, the surrounding inflammation and edema in the soft tissues make visualization difficult and cause discomfort for the patient. Studies are immediately obtained if re-established pulses are lost, become equivocal and/or symptoms of ischemia occur. Autogenous grafts are typically studied at the first follow-up visit to establish a baseline. Then studies are obtained at 3-month intervals during the first year, 6-month intervals during the second year and annually thereafter. Synthetic grafts may be studied if there is a change in ABI or patient symptomatology. High-risk synthetic grafts performed for limb salvage in the absence of an autogenous conduit are studied similarly to autogenous grafts.

A significant decrease in ABI and/or change in flow velocity has been reported to be predictive of early graft failure. A decrease in the ABI of 0.15–0.20 and a peak systolic flow velocity >200 cm/s, or flow velocities <45 cm/s, are indicative of a graft stenosis of 50% or better. Early intervention by angioplasty, reoperation or a combination of these modalities has been shown significantly to improve assisted primary and secondary patency rates of grafts [39-41]. The assisted primary patency rate of a graft refers to any graft that is intervened upon by treatment of an anatomical abnormality to maintain patency prior to impending occlusion. Secondary patency refers to opening an occluded graft to reestablish flow.

Diabetic considerations

Diabetes is a significant risk factor for the development of PAD. The likelihood of developing soft tissue gangrene is 50 times greater for the diabetic patient versus the nondiabetic patient. This is thought to be secondary to the interrelated factors of diabetic neuropathy (sensory and motor deficits in the foot) and increased pressure on the plantar metatarsal heads, secondary to atrophy of the intrinsic muscles of the foot, in combination with compromised circulation.

Anatomic distribution of arterial lesions in diabetics is somewhat different from that of nondiabetics; however, the underlying histopathology is similar. Diabetic arterial disease is more common in the distal profunda femoris artery, distal popliteal artery, tibial artery and digital arteries of the foot. The aortoiliac arteries are frequently not involved. These patients tend to develop intimal thickening in addition to the primary pathology of atherosclerosis in large vessels. Noninvasive ankle-brachial studies may be inconclusive owing to significant calcification of the vessel media rendering the vasculature noncompressible.

Management should be centered around prompt evaluation and treatment of any infection with broad spectrum antimicrobial agents, and surgical debridement if needed [42]. Prior to any surgical debridement, standard foot films should be obtained and may provide an insight into bony involvement. This may necessarily alter the operative plan [43]. Standard vascular evaluation and treatment of disease progresses along the same pathways as described above with attention to correction of hemodynamically significant lesions for limb salvage.

Amputation

Unfortunately, amputations secondary to vascular disease do occur. In situations where there are no bypass options and the infectious risk of gangrenous tissue or the pain outweighs the surgical risk, amputation is indicated.

Patients who present with rest pain, tissue loss and gangrene should be evaluated for bypass based upon current function. For example, the patient who was ambulating and self-sufficient with an independent lifestyle prior to onset of ischemia and infection would certainly be different from the patient who was bed-bound and dependent.

However, regardless of functional status, the patient must have a distal blood vessel with which to construct a vascular surgical bypass to have any hope of success. If reconstruction is not an option based upon the discussed criteria then intervention, i.e. amputation, should be carried out when infectious complications necessitate, or the patient's pain can no longer be controlled with reasonable pharmacologic means. The amputation should be performed at the level that will provide adequate blood supply for healing.

Summary

Peripheral arterial disease is becoming increasingly more prevalent and will continue to increase as life expectancy lengthens and the elderly population grows. Prompt recognition of potentially limb threatening conditions and early intervention or vascular consultation are instrumental to limb salvage and overall morbidity and mortality. The choice of conduit for bypass has been shown to have a significant impact on overall graft patency rates with autogenous vein providing the best results. Additionally, graft surveillance and aggressive intervention has been shown to improve overall graft salvage rates. Finally, if no anatomical options exist for surgical bypass then the risk of infectious complications and chronic pain must be taken into consideration and amputation should be considered.

References

1. Wilt TJ. Current strategies in the diagnosis and management of lower extremity peripheral vascular disease. J Gen Intern Med 1992;**7**(1):87–101.

2. Gardner AW, Poehlman ET. Exercise rehabilitation programs for the treatment of intermittent claudication pain: a meta analysis. JAMA 1995;**274**(12):975–80.

3. Regensteiner JG. Assessing ambulation, functional status, and quality of life in patients with claudication. Am J Med June 1999:16–22.

4. Hiatt WR, Regensteiner JG, Hargarten ME et al. Benefit of exercise conditioning for patients with peripheral arterial disease. Circulation 1990;**81**(2):60–59.

5. Hertzer N. Surgical management of intermittent claudication. Am Fam Physician 1997;**16**(3):108–16.

6. Brewster DC. Clinical and anatomical considerations for surgery in aortoiliac disease and results of surgical treatment. Circulation 1991;**83**(2 Suppl.):I-425I–52.

7. Rutherford RB. Options in the surgical management of aorto-iliac occlusive disease: a changing perspective. Cardiovasc Surg 1999;**7**(1):5–12.

8. Brewster DC. Current controversies in the management of aortoiliac occlusive disease. J Vasc Surg 1997;**25**(2):365–79.

9. Whiteley MS, Ray-Chaudhuri SB, Galland RB. Changing patterns in aortoiliac reconstruction: a 7-year audit. *Br J Surg* 1996;**83**(10):1367–9.

10. Sullivan TM, Childs MB, Bacharach JM et al. Percutaneous transluminal angioplasty and primary stenting of the iliac arteries in 288 patients. *J Vasc Surg* 1997;**25**(5):829–39.

11. Bosch JL, Hunink MG. Meta-analysis of the results of percutaneous transluminal angioplasty and stent placement for aortoiliac occlusive disease. *Radiology* 1997;**204**(1):87–96.

12. Ballard JL, Bergan JJ, Singh P et al. Aortoiliac stent deployment versus surgical reconstruction: analysis of outcome and cost. *J Vasc Surg* 1998;**28**(1):94–103.

13. Szilagyi DE, Elliott JP, Smith RF, et al: A thirty year survery of the reconstructive surgical Treatment of aortoiliac occlusive disease. *J Vasc Surg* 1986;**3**(3):421–36.

14. de Vries SO, Hunink MG. Results of aortic bifurcation grafts for aortoiliac occlusive disease: a meta-analysis. *J Vasc Surg* 1997;**26**(4):558–69.

15. Passman MA, Taylor LM, Moneta GL et al: Comparison of axillofemoral and aortofemoral bypass for aortoiliac occlusive disease. *J Vasc Surg* 1996;**23**(2):263–71.

16. Meister RH, Schweiger H, Lang W. Knitted double-velour Dacron prostheses in aortobifemoral position — long-term performance of different coating materials. *Vasa* 1998;**27**(4):236–9.

17. Polterauer P, Prager M, Holzenbein T et al. Dacron versus polytetrafluoroethylene for Y-aortic bifucation grafts: a six year prospective, randomized trial. *Surgery* 1992;**111**(6):626–33.

18. Brombacher GD, Van Marle J. Importance of the profunda femoral artery in distal limb revascularisation. *S Afr J Surg* 1997;**35**(4):185–7.

19. Cron JP, Blanchard D, Baud F et al. Long-term of patients receiving an aorto-bi-femoral prosthesis for atherosclerotic occlusive disease of the aortic bifurcation. *Int Angiol* 1994;**13**(4):300–7.

20. Prendiville EJ, Burke PE, Colgan MP et al. The profunda femoris: a durable outflow vessel in aortofemoral surgery. *J Vasc Surg* 1992;**16**(1):23–9.

21. Poulias GE, Doundoulakis N, Prombonas E et al. Aorto-femoral bypass and determinants of early success and late favourable outcome: experience with 1000 consecutive cases. *J Cardiovasc Surg (Torino)* 1992;**33**(6):664–78.

22. McKinsey JF. Exta-anatomic reconstruction. *Surg Clin North Am* 1995;**75**(4):731–40.

23. Biancari F, Lepantalo M. Extra-anatomic bypass surgery for critical leg ischemia: a review. *J Cardiovasc Surg (Torino)* 1998;**39**(3):295–301.

24. Johnson WC, Lee KK. Comparative evaluation of externally supported dacron and polytetrafluoroethylene prosthetic bypasses for femorofemoral and axillofemoral arterial reconstructions. Veterans Affairs Cooperative Study #141. *J Vasc Surg* 1999;**30**(6):1077–83.

25. Schneider JR, Besso SR, Walsh DB et al. Femorofemoral versus aortobifemoral bypass: Outcome And hemodynamic results. *J Vasc Surg* 1994;**19**(1):435–7.

26. Schneider JR, McDaniel MD, Walsh DB et al. Axillofemoral bypass: outcome and hemodynamic results in high-risk patients. *J Vasc Surg* 1992;**15**(6):952–63.

27. Harrington ME, Harrington EB, Haimov M et al. Axillogemoral bypass: compromised bypass for compromised patients. *J Vasc Surg* 1994;**20**(2):195–201.

28. Illig KA, Green RM. Prosthetic above-knee femoropopliteal bypass. *Semin Vasc Surg* 1999;**12**(1):38–45.

29. Belkin M, Knox J, Donaldson MC et al. Infrainguinal arterial reconstruction with nonreversed greater saphenous vein. *J Vasc Surg* 1996;**24**(6):957–62.

30. Shah DM, Darling C, Chang BB et al. Long-term results of in-situ saphenous vein bypass. Analysis of 2058 cases. *Ann Surg* 1995;**222**(4):438–48.

31. Abbott WM, Green RM, Matsumoto T et al. Prosthetic above-knee femoropopliteal bypass grafting: results of a multicenter randomized prospective trial. Above-Knee Femoropopliteal Study Group. *J Vasc Surg* 1997;**25**(1):19–28.

32. Verhelst R, Bruneau M, Nicolas AL et al. Popliteal-to-distal bypass grafts for limb salvage. *Ann Vasc Surg* 1997;**11**(5):50–59.

33. Veith FJ, Gupta SK, Ascer E et al. Six-year prospective multicenter randomized comparison of autologous saphenous vein and expanded polytetrafluoroethylene grafts in infrainguinal arterial reconstructions. *J Vasc Surg* 1986;**3**(1):104–14.

34. Comparative evaluation of reversed, and in situ vein bypass grafts in distal popliteal and tibial-peroneal revascularization. Veteran Administration Study Group 141. *Arch Surg* 1988;**123**(4):434–8.

35. Whittemore AD, Belkin M: Infrainguinal Bypass. In: Rutherford *Vascular Surgery*. 5th Ed. Philadelphia, PA:WB Saunders & Co, 2000: 998–1018.

36. Hansen AK, Bille S, Nielson PH et al. Profundaplasty as the only reconstructive procedure in patients with severe ischemia of the lower extremity. *Surg Gynecol Obstet* 1990;**171**(1):47–50.

37. Jacobs DL, Seabrook GR, Freischlag JA et al. The current role of profundaplasty in complex arterial reconstruction. *Vasc Surg* 1995;**29**.

38. Harward TR, Ingegno MD, Carlton L et al. Limb-threatening ischemia due to multilevel arterial occlusive disease. *Ann Surg* 1995;**221**(5):4985–06.

39. Lundell A, Lindblad B, Bergqvist D et al: Femoropopliteal-crural graft patency is improved by an intensive surveillance program: A prospective randomized study. *J Vasc Surg* 1995;**21**(1):26–34.

40. Mattos MA, van Bemmelen PS, Hodgson K et al. Does correction of stenoses identified with color duplex improve infrainguinal graft patency? *J Vasc Surg* 1993;**17**(1):54–66.

41. Gentile AT, Mills JL, Gooden MA et al. Identification of predictors for lower extremity vein graft stenosis. *Am J Surg* 1997;**174**(2):218–21.

42. Steed DL, Donohoe D, Webster MW. Effect of extensive debridement and treatment of the healing of diabetic foot ulcers. Diabetic Ulcer Study Group. *J Am Coll Surg* 1996;**183**(1):61–4.

43. Longmaid HE, Kruskal JB. Imaging infections in diabetic patients. *Infect Dis Clin North Am* 1995;**9**(1):163–81.

chapter six

Endovascular Intervention

Kenneth Rosenfield and Mandeep Dhadly

Introduction

It has been 35 years since the landmark event in 1964 when Dotter and Judkins published their original report of a peripheral arterial recanalization [1]. Currently, atherosclerotic peripheral arterial disease (PAD) is estimated to be present in more than 20% of people over the age of 65 years, and the prevalence of this disease will probably increase with the aging demographics of the population. Therapy of PAD has historically rested in the domain of the vascular surgeon, and has primarily involved endarterectomy or bypass procedures. These operations commonly require general anesthesia and involve significant blood loss and fluid shifts, in a patient population with frequent co-morbidities including major cardiac, pulmonary and renal disease. Rehabilitation following such procedures may be prolonged. When it is possible to provide a similar level of correction and durability of benefit with catheter-based (i.e. endovascular) treatments, risk and disability may be minimized. Significant technological advances in imaging and equipment, particularly over the past 10 years, have enabled safer and more effective endovascular therapy for PAD. Recent validation of these endovascular techniques in specific clinical situations based on results from clinical trials, as well as the availability of superior tools, has fueled a relative explosion in the field of peripheral endovascular intervention.

Endovascular intervention for peripheral arterial disease

Endovascular therapy in the peripheral vascular system shares the same heritage as coronary intervention through the pioneering work of Dotter, Judkins, Gruentzig and others [1,2]. In fact, most of the techniques now used in the coronaries (e.g. balloon dilatation, stenting and atherectomy) were first employed in the peripheral circulation. Recent innovations that have made such therapies safer and more effective include improvements in catheter, guidewire and balloon design, and the availability of endovascular stents. Guidewires and catheters with small diameters, 'torquability', 'steerability' and atraumatic tips are available, often with lubricious coatings to enhance passage. Balloons are now chiefly constructed of high tensile strength, ultra-thin wall polymers, allowing selection based on a list of characteristics including compliance curves, profile, 'pushability', re-wrap and stent retention. With these advances, intervention in virtually all major diseased vessels in the peripheral circulation is now possible. Finally, progressive advances have been made in stent design since the prototypical Palmaz (balloon-expandable) and Wallstent (self-expandable) models, increasing ease of deliverability to the target site, conformability to the vessel contour, radial support, visibility and side-branch access. Outcome has also been improved by innovations and improvements in imaging techniques, such as digital enhancement of conventional contrast images and intravascular ultrasound (IVUS). The latter provides a cross-sectional view of the vessel similar to a histologic section, and better comprehension of the mechanisms responsible for successful angioplasty.

When catheter-based therapy is possible, it is attractive to patients, providers and insurers, since it can usually be performed as a cost-saving 'same-day' procedure with low morbidity and rapid convalescence. Even in instances where the degree of revascularization is not as complete, or where symptomatic improvement may not be as durable, the reduced morbidity of a catheter-based therapy may make it attractive in high-risk patients. The availability of effective, less invasive percutaneous options for revascularization has also led to a re-evaluation and reduction of the threshold for intervention. For example, a patient whose claudication is not severe enough to warrant major surgical bypass may nonetheless be appropriate for percutaneous transluminal angioplasty (PTA). Most therapeutic decisions should be made by trained vascular specialists, preferably working collaboratively in multidisciplinary teams composed of vascular surgeons, radiologists and cardiologists.

The current recommendations for revascularization at various peripheral sites are summarized in Table 1. Since therapy for many sites is evolving

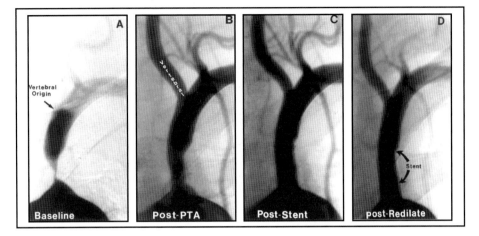

Figure 1. PTA-stenting of subclavian artery stenosis with associated subclavian steal syndrome. A. Baseline angiogram depicts critical stenosis at origin of left subclavian artery. Vertebral artery is not visualized secondary to retrograde flow which also has the effect of diluting the contrast in the subclavian artery distal to the vertebral artery origin. B. Post-PTA with a 7 mm balloon. Antegrade flow is now restored in the vertebral artery but there is significant recoil of plaque at the lesion site. C. Palmaz stent deployed with an 8 mm balloon, lumen enlarged; minor irregularities seen along border of stent. D. Post-redilation with 9 mm balloon.

rapidly, vascular specialists must have a comprehensive understanding of all aspects of a given revascularization procedure including:

1. the indications for intervention

2. the therapeutic alternatives available and their expected outcomes

3. the techniques employed during an intervention

4. the potential complications

Subclavian and innominate arteries

Clinical indications for subclavian PTA include symptomatic ischemia of the posterior fossa and/or upper extremities, with or without subclavian steal syndrome, and functional preservation of the internal mammary conduit in the setting of coronary artery bypass grafting (CABG) (Figure 1). While no randomized trials exist comparing surgery and PTA for subclavian disease, PTA is now considered the first line therapy for focal subclavian stenoses, since most published series of subclavian PTA report technical success of >90% and complication rates of <10% [3-5]. Stenting may further improve the results, as recent series using primary stenting indicate [6-8]. If the lesion is adjacent to, or spans, the origins of the vertebral artery and/or internal mammary artery (IMA), attempts should be made to avoid placing these vessels into 'stent jail' (occurring when the stent struts block side branches of arteries and complicate future treatment). Most left subclavian lesions are located proximal to the vertebral artery, where the use of either balloon-expandable or self-expanding stents is reasonable. For lesions located beyond the IMA, self-expanding stents should be used to avoid the potential for stent compression by extravascular structures at the thoracic outlet.

Complications are generally minor and infrequent, but may include problems at the femoral or brachial access site, as well as inadvertent 'jailing', dissection or embolization of the vertebral artery or left internal mammary artery (LIMA) [9]. Recurrence rates are low (5–10%), and may be treated by stenting (if not stented initially) or balloon angioplasty (for in-stent restenosis). Treatment of occlusive subclavian disease is more controversial since PTA is associated with a lower chance of success (50–75%) and an increased risk of embolization of thrombus or atheroma into the cerebral, upper extremity or coronary circulations.

Carotid arteries

Atherosclerotic disease occurs predominantly at the common carotid bifurcation, a site that is conveniently accessible for surgical carotid endarterectomy (CEA). Stenosis at the origin or proximal aspect of the common carotid artery is less common, and surgical treatment may involve a thoracotomy or subclavian-carotid bypass. The landmark NASCET (North American Symptomatic Carotid Endarterectomy Trial) and ACAS trials demonstrated that surgical endarterectomy, when performed for carotid bifurcation disease by experienced vascular surgeons on appropriately selected patients, is effective in reducing the likelihood of stroke compared to medical therapy[10,11]. Accordingly, percutaneous treatment of carotid arteries has thus far been reserved for circumstances where the surgical risk is considered high or excessive (Figure 2) [12-14].

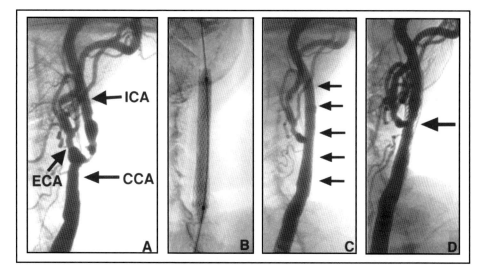

Figure 2. PTA-stenting of left carotid artery in a patient deemed high risk for surgery because of prior neck surgery and radiation therapy for carcinoma of the tongue, and who also had left carotid endarterectomy one year ago. A. Baseline angiography reveals restenosis at the origin of the internal carotid artery (ICA). Non-obstructive atherosclerotic disease is present in the common carotid (CCA) and external carotid (ECA). B. After deployment of a 20 mm self-expanding Wallstent, post-dilation is performed with a 5 mm balloon. C. There is an excellent final angiographic result, and the stent is well expanded (arrows). D. Follow-up angiography at 9 months with the stent widely patent and mild focal in-stent restenosis (arrow).

Primary (as opposed to provisional) stenting confers an advantage over PTA, and favorable intermediate-term results are now available [15-17], suggesting safety and efficacy comparable to CEA. In Roubin's update as of May 1999 (personal communication), a total of 482 patients (569 vessels) underwent elective stent placement over a 5-year period. Approximately 40% had symptomatic cerebral ischemia and 80% had severe coronary artery disease (CAD). Higher risk anatomical features included contralateral occlusion (10%), prior ipsilateral CEA (17%) and many causes of unfavorable surgical anatomy. Despite these challenges, the technical success was 98%, and acute (30-day) results were similar to CEA for this high risk cohort: 8 patients (1.6%) died (half not related to the procedure); 4 (0.8%) had major cerebrovascular accidents (CVA); and 29 (5.1%) had minor, non-disabling stroke (lasting >24 h but resolved by 30 days). Based on the successful outcomes from this and other smaller series prospective randomized studies have been initiated to compare the percutaneous versus surgical modalities in both high-risk (Stenting and Angioplasty with Protection in Patients at High-Risk for Endarterectomy — the SAPPHIRE trial) and average-risk (Carotid Revascularization Endarterectomy versus Stent Trial — CREST) surgical candidates.

It remains to be determined what is the best stent design for use in the carotid arteries. Although balloon-expandable Palmaz biliary stents were used initially by many groups, the infrequent but troublesome occurrence of stent compression [18] has led most investigators to favor the use of self-expanding stents at the carotid bifurcation. Most investigators agree that the future of carotid stenting will probably employ nitinol, self-expanding stents, that are lower profile, 0.014/0.018-inch based and able to be placed accurately. Additionally, there is tremendous enthusiasm surrounding the development of distal protection devices, both balloon occlusion and filter types, to avoid cerebral embolization during carotid angioplasty. It is anticipated that these may significantly reduce the embolic complications associated with carotid PTA and stenting.

Renal arteries

Renal artery stenosis (RAS) is a common manifestation of generalized atherosclerosis that tends to be under-diagnosed and under-treated. It has been estimated to be the cause of 10–20% of new-onset end-stage renal disease in individuals over 50 years of age [19]. The primary goals of renal artery revascularization are to improve control of hypertension, preserve or restore renal function, and treat other potential adverse physiologic effects of severe renal artery stenosis (e.g. congestive heart failure, recurrent flash pulmonary edema and angina) [20,21]. When analyzing indications and results, it is important to distinguish between the two major etiologies of renal artery stenosis: fibromuscular dysplasia (FMD) and the more common atherosclerotic disease.

Fibromuscular dysplasia

When FMD is localized within the main renal artery or its primary branches, it can be treated quite effectively with balloon angioplasty alone [22]. Initial technical success exceeds 90%, and initial clinical success (elimination or significant reduction in hypertension at 6-month follow-up) is roughly 85%, with a 5-year recurrence rate under 10%. However, FMD that involves multiple distal branch vessels and/or aneurysmal disease is better treated surgically.

Atherosclerotic renal artery stenosis

During the 1980s, balloon angioplasty proved to be a safe and effective modality, but one with a restenosis rate that approached 70% at 6–12 months. This previously served as a compelling reason to recommend primary surgical revascularization in patients who were good surgical candidates, despite an associated mortality of 2–17% [23]. In the 1990s, however, numerous investigators have demonstrated more complete amelioration of the stenosis and trans-stenotic pressure gradient following stent deployment in aorto-ostial lesions, with a lower restenosis rate, compared to balloon angioplasty alone (Figure 3). Palmaz [21], in a recent position paper, summarized the results of stenting in 349 patients from eight series, followed for a mean duration of 10.9 months. Hypertension was improved in 56% and cured in 10%; and renal function improved in 27% and stabilized in 38%. Restenosis occurred in approximately 16% of patients, with major complications in 4.9%, although these were reduced in the more recent series.

There remains great controversy regarding the indication, timing, method, risk and benefit of renal artery revascularization. Many patients who undergo renal artery revascularization fail to demonstrate any significant clinical response. For patients with hypertension, the following clinical factors are predictive of a successful outcome:

1. rapid acceleration of hypertension over a number of weeks or months, where blood pressure was previously well controlled on a stable medical regimen
2. presence of 'malignant' hypertension
3. hypertension in association with flash pulmonary edema
4. contemporaneous rapid rise in creatinine
5. development of azotemia in response to ACE inhibitors

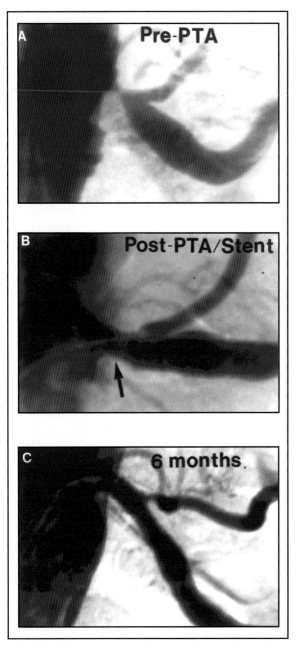

Figure 3. Prophylactic renal artery revascularization prior to coronary artery bypass surgery (CABG). Patient with unstable angina and three-vessel coronary artery disease requiring semi-urgent CABG. Hypertension had recently accelerated (SBP >200 mm Hg) and renal function had deteriorated.
A. Baseline renal angiogram performed at the same time as cardiac catheterization demonstrated occlusion of the right renal artery and 99% stenosis in the left renal artery. B. Angiogram immediately following PTA-stent (arrow) deployment shows restoration of lumen. Blood pressure normalized, and the patient subsequently had an uneventful CABG.
C. Renal angiogram 6 months post-PTA demonstrates widely patent stent site.

For salvage or preservation of renal function, those with a recent rapid rise in creatinine (unexplained) by other factors, azotemia resulting from ACE inhibitors, and absence of diabetes or other causes of intrinsic kidney disease have the best response. Conversely, patients with severe baseline renal insufficiency secondary to nephrosclerosis (e.g. diabetic nephropathy) with superimposed RAS but minimal trans-stenotic pressure gradient, or a kidney shrunken to less than 8 cm in length, are unlikely to benefit from renal artery intervention. In cases of doubt about severity, trans-stenotic pressure gradients should be measured at the time of intervention. A gradient of mean blood pressure in excess of 10 mmHg and/or systolic blood pressure in excess of 20 mmHg is considered significant. Below this level of gradient, a patient is unlikely to benefit dramatically with respect to blood pressure control or renal function, although an argument could be made to treat patients in order to prevent progression of disease.

Complications

Complications related to balloon angioplasty and/or stenting of renal arteries occur in less than 10% of patients and most commonly involve access. The most feared complication, however, is that of atheroembolism either into the renal or peripheral vascular bed. To minimize this risk, aggressive manipulation of catheters should be avoided. The signs of cholesterol embolization include persistent hypertension despite successful renal artery revascularization, gradual rise in creatinine over the succeeding weeks or months, the presence of livido reticularis on the abdominal wall or in the lower extremities, and the presence of eosinophilia on a peripheral blood smear. There is no known effective treatment for the renal manifestations of cholesterol embolization once it occurs; however, some have reported the effective resolution of lower extremity rest pain and ulceration using IV prostaglandin [24]. Other complications of percutaneous renal revascularization include dissection of the renal artery or the wall of the aorta, acute or delayed thrombosis, stent embolization, infection and rupture of the renal artery.

Aortoiliac obstructive disease

While balloon dilatation has been applied to atherosclerotic disease at every site in the body, nowhere have the results been superior to those achieved in the aortoiliac vessels. Aortoiliac revascularization is currently recommended for four indications:

1. relief of symptomatic lower extremity ischemia, including claudication, rest pain, ulceration or gangrene

2. restoration and/or preservation of inflow to the lower extremity in the setting of preexisting or anticipated distal bypass

3. procurement of access to more proximal vascular beds for anticipated invasive procedures (e.g. cardiac catheterization/percutaneous transluminal coronary angioplasty [PTCA] or intra-aortic balloon insertion)

4. occasionally, to rescue flow-limiting dissection complicating access for other invasive procedures (Figure 4)

Aorto-bifemoral bypass has a long-term patency of 90% at one year, 75–80% at five years and 60–70% at ten years, but carries a mortality of between 2 and 3%. Accordingly, surgical intervention has been reserved for patients with critical limb ischemia or advanced degrees of disability. Because percutaneous angioplasty is less invasive, has fewer complications and a lower cost, the threshold at which intervention is offered to patients with aorto-iliac disease may be lower [25].

Most atherosclerotic aortic disease extends into the iliac arteries, and requires dilation of both territories. In fact revascularization at the aortic bifurcation commonly utilizes either 'kissing balloons' or 'kissing stents' (Figure 5) [26]. The results of balloon angioplasty alone for iliac *stenoses*, particularly focal lesions, are excellent, with acute technical and clinical success in excess of 90%, based on a large number of reports [27,28]. One-, three- and five-year patencies range from approximately 75–95%, 60–90% and 55–85%, respectively. Factors associated with good results

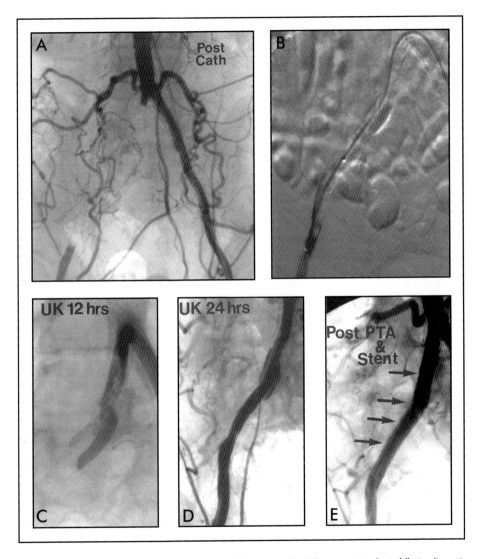

Figure 4. Thrombolysis, PTA and stent deployment in a patient with acute onset of right lower extremity ischemia following diagnostic cardiac catheterization. A. Baseline arteriogram reveals fresh thrombotic occlusion of right common iliac artery, with reconstitution of common femoral artery by collaterals. B. Occlusion is crossed in antegrade fashion from contralateral side, and infusion of urokinase (UK) is begun via Mewissen catheter. C. Following 12 hours of UK, the common and external iliac arteries are now partially patent but have extensive dissection, residual thrombus and blind cul-de-sac. Thrombolytic therapy is therefore continued. D. Following 24 hours of UK, the vessel is now patent and thrombus resolved, but extensive dissection remains. E. Following deployment of two Palmaz stents, the iliac artery is widely patent, with amelioration of dissection and elimination of the cul-de-sac. The patient remains asymptomatic four years later.

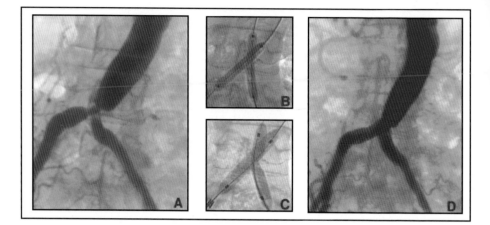

Figure 5. PTA and 'kissing stents' deployment for aorto-iliac bifurcation disease in a patient with bilateral severe limb claudication. A. Baseline angiogram demonstrates severe atherosclerotic stenosis of the terminal aorta, extending into both common iliac arteries. B. After obtaining arterial access from both sides of the groin, PTA is performed with simultaneously inflated ('kissing') 6 mm balloons. C. Two 38 mm long HercuLink stents are deployed on 9 mm balloons at 10 atm. D. Both iliac arteries are widely patent, although there is mild residual stenosis in the distal aorta. The patient is asymptomatic at 6 month follow-up.

include: focal lesion; large vessel size; common iliac (as opposed to external iliac); single lesion (as opposed to multiple serial lesions); male gender; lesser Rutherford category (claudication as opposed to critical limb ischemia); and presence of good runoff. The results in patients with total occlusion, diffuse disease, smaller vessels, diabetes mellitus, female gender, critical limb ischemia and poor runoff are less favorable.

Using stents, acute technical success is in the range of 95–100%, with an average 1-year patency of 90%, and an average 3-year patency of 75% [29]. Because of superior cosmetic and hemodynamic results, a strategy of primary stent deployment for aortoiliac vessels has been adopted by many interventionists, though others reserve stenting only for suboptimal angioplasty results. A meta-analysis performed by Bosch et al. [28] on 14 recent studies (all published after 1990), involving more than 2100 patients undergoing aortoiliac PTA, revealed a higher immediate success rate for stents than for PTA alone (96 vs. 91%), with a subsequent 4-year primary patency rate of 77% for stenting versus 65% for PTA alone.

Complications with aortoiliac angioplasty are relatively infrequent (<6% based upon multiple series). Most common are access site complications, including local or retroperitoneal bleeding, pseudoaneurysm and arteriovenous (AV) fistula. Retroperitoneal bleeding can occasionally be fatal if not controlled. Arterial rupture is rare, but must be recognized promptly and controlled by inflation of a balloon within the lesion (balloon tamponade), reversal of anticoagulation and volume resuscitation. Surgical repair may be required, although stent-grafts are in development, and could potentially be used to treat this complication. Distal embolization occurs in less than 5% [25].

Abdominal aortic aneurysm

The endovascular repair of abdominal aortic aneurysms using stent grafts represents one of the most dramatic advances in the less invasive treatment of vascular disease. Although this field is still in its infancy, great strides have been made with the devices and technology so that the many patients with abdominal aortic aneurysmal disease requiring repair would probably qualify anatomically for one of the available devices. While the current gold standard for treatment of this disorder remains open surgical repair, a substantial number of patients who have aneurysms ≥ 5 cm in diameter are not deemed to be candidates for surgery due to unsuitable anatomy or the presence of co-morbid conditions. The prognosis is grim for these patients, as described by Perko et al. [30]. Of the 170 patients deemed inoperable, 132 (78%) died during the period of the study; 78 (59%) died specifically from rupture. For those who are surgical candidates, the operative mortality of aneurysm resection is between 1.4 and 7.6% [31], but increases substantially for those whose aneurysms are symptomatic. The potential for endovascular stent-grafts to lower the morbidity and mortality in these high-risk or inoperable patients has provided a compelling reason to pursue the development of these devices. The first stent-graft procedure in a human was performed by Parodi in Argentina [32], who implanted a straight Dacron tube graft affixed at its proximal end to a large balloon-expandable Palmaz stent. A distal stent was subsequently added to the device to control retrograde flow into the aneurysm sac (endoleak). Several stent grafts have since been developed and subjected to clinical trials; two of these (the AneuRx and EVT devices) received FDA approval in 1999 and are now commercially available.

More than 5000 stent-graft procedures for abdominal aortic aneurysm exclusion have been performed worldwide. Recently published series describe the multicenter prospective experience with the AneuRx stent-graft [33] and the Boston Scientific Vanguard [31] devices. Both demonstrate success rates approaching 90%, endoleaks in about 10% and reduction in morbidity compared to conventional repair, but have a steep learning curve that entails mastering device and patient selection issues. Aneurysms with a short or absent proximal neck (distance between the lower border of the renal artery and the beginning of the aneurysm) are more difficult to treat, although some device iterations now incorporate additional bare stent material designed to be deployed proximally overlying the renal vessels, with the graft material beginning just below the renal arteries. Other issues remain, such as the large caliber (18–28 French) of the current devices.

Lower extremity

Superficial femoral and popliteal arteries

Decisions regarding intervention, whether surgery or PTA, for infra-inguinal disease must take into account the degree to which the patient is disabled, the presence of co-morbid factors and the anticipated short- and long-term outcome. In general, patients with mild, non-disabling claudication should *not* undergo interventional therapy for superficial femoral (SFA) disease, but rather should be placed on conservative treatment with an exercise program.

There remains considerable controversy as to the relative role of percutaneous therapy versus surgery. In a recent review, Murray and colleagues [34] noted that the technical success of PTA improved from 70% to 91% between 1980 and 1989 with excellent acute and long-term efficacy, even for lesions greater than 10 cm in length. Similarly, the success rate in crossing *occluded* segments of the SFA and popliteal artery has improved dramatically, probably as a consequence of technical advances. Foremost among these is the use of hydrophilic guidewires. Among several large series of patients undergoing PTA of femoral-popliteal stenoses and occlusions, the majority of whom were claudicants, the acute technical success was between 82% and 96% [35-38]. Primary patency rates at one, three and five years averaged approximately 60%, 50% and 45%, respectively. Several factors influence long-term outcome following SFA/popliteal angioplasty. Patients with intermittent claudication (versus tissue loss), a more severe lesion at baseline and lower post-treatment residual stenosis tend to have a *better* outcome at one year; those with diabetes, threatened limb loss or diffuse atherosclerotic vascular disease with zero to one vessel runoff, have a worse outcome.

For stenoses of the SFA and popliteal artery, the standard approach is that of balloon angioplasty. In contrast to the documented benefits achieved by the use of endovascular stents for iliac PTA, experience thus far in the SFA has been less favorable. Therefore, at present, SFA/popliteal stenting should be limited to cases of flow-limiting dissection or clearly failed PTA. Some promising strategies have emerged on the horizon for treating the vexing problem of SFA restenosis. Firstly, endovascular brachytherapy, which is currently being tested in coronary arteries, is also undergoing study in conjunction with SFA/popliteal PTA. Similarly, it is hoped that covered stents or local drug delivery might reduce the incidence of restenosis. In limb salvage situations where direct arterial recanalization is impossible, creation of new collaterals using genetic material has been termed 'therapeutic angiogenesis' [39-41]. This approach appears to hold great promise.

Infra-popliteal arteries

As technological advances have been made, including the development of low-profile balloons and atraumatic coronary guidewires, the ability to treat infrapopliteal disease has improved. Over the past decade, since Schwarten and colleagues [42] reported the first sizable series of patients undergoing infrapopliteal revascularization, the application of these techniques has become more widespread. Infrapopliteal stenoses and occlusions can be revascularized percutaneously with remarkably low risk and technical success rates in the range of 80–95%. In one recent large series reported by Dorros et al. [43], success was achieved in 406/417 patients (96%); success rate in stenoses (98%) was superior to that in occlusions (76%). In-hospital complications were extremely low. Although follow-up is incomplete, the vast majority of patients with critical limb ischemia (95%) improved following revascularization. Such improvement does not necessarily imply ongoing patency. Restoration of flow through only one of the three major vessels to the foot may be sufficient to heal a distal ischemic lesion, and, once healed, most patients will do well even in the face of documented reocclusion or restenosis.

Although balloon angioplasty alone is the conventional approach, rotational atherectomy or excimer laser angioplasty can be useful as adjunctive therapy. Specifically, lesions that have unfavorable morphology, such as total occlusions, heavy calcification and ostial disease, may benefit from these 'niche' devices [44,45].

Many of the patients treated with infra-popliteal angioplasty to date have been those who were too high-risk or otherwise unqualified for bypass surgery [46]. The latter is still considered to be the standard of care for patients with critical limb ischemia due to infra-popliteal disease. Regardless of the conduit used (reversed vein, *in situ* vein or prosthetic material), patency rates are inferior to those of more proximal reconstruction. It is conceivable that the long-term clinical outcome of percutaneous therapy may ultimately equal that of distal bypass grafting. A randomized controlled trial will be required to address this issue. It is also conceivable that both of these revascularization strategies will be replaced in many instances by the strategy of therapeutic angiogenesis [47]. If the body can be stimulated to create its own new microcirculation, then the issues of restenosis, reocclusion and graft closure become moot.

Lower extremity bypass grafts

Graft failure, or impending graft failure, is often not heralded by increasing clinical symptoms. Accordingly, a strategy of regular graft surveillance using duplex ultrasonography is recommended in order to preserve and extend the life of the graft. For impending graft failure, either detected by duplex ultrasonography or increasing symptoms, immediate arteriography is recommended, followed by either surgical or percutaneous revascularization. Focal lesions of the proximal or distal anastomosis, anastomoses or short-segment lesions (3 cm or less) occurring within the bypass graft are amenable to PTA [25]. Lengthy lesions (especially more than 10 cm) and stenoses associated with anastomotic aneurysms are recommended for surgical revision.

Thrombolytic therapy

For occlusions in peripheral vessels or lower extremity bypass grafts, catheter-directed thrombolysis is much more effective than systemic fibrinolysis. The technical aspects of use vary among investigators. There is agreement that the catheter must penetrate into the occlusion in order for the lytic agent to have any effect. Some prefer going one step further and crossing the occlusion primarily, in order to 'lace' the lytic agent throughout the occlusion and enhance the efficiency of thrombolysis. Urokinase has previously been the agent of choice, with alternatives of tPA [48] and Retavase. Other catheter-based therapies include the AngioJet rheolytic thrombectomy device, which efficiently removes fresh thrombus, as well as that partially degraded by thrombolytic agents.

Summary

Advances in technology, together with supportive evidence from clinical studies, have led to a paradigm shift in our approach to the management of peripheral arterial disease. The availability of safer and more effective techniques has lowered the threshold for intervention in a field where the only alternative to a major surgical procedure has often meant ongoing pain and/or morbidity. Further refinement of endovascular techniques, along with enhanced evaluation and recognition of atherosclerotic vascular disease, promises to make peripheral endovascular intervention a major growth area over the next decade.

TABLE 1. Revascularization strategy for various locations (as of 2/00).

Arterial site and lesion type	Revascularization strategy					Clinical indication (e.g. Rutherford category/other)*	
	Percutaneous				Surgery	Percutaneous	Surgery
	Balloon angioplasty (PTA)	Stent	Adjunctive therapy				
			Thrombolysis	Other			
Brachiocephalic vessels							
Subclavian stenosis/ occlusion	Preferred treatment for stenosis. Successful in most occlusions	Not approved; stents useful to optimize PTA results	Indicated for recent occlusion (<1 month). May facilitate PTA in chronic occlusion, but little published experience		Reserved for PTA non-candidates or failures who have severe symptoms	Moderate arm claudication, subclavian steal syndrome, coronary steal syndrome or coronary steal via internal mammary artery	Severe arm claudication and/or subclavian steal syndrome
Carotid							
A. Innominate and common carotid (intrathoracic)	Preferred therapy for patients with symptoms or asymptomatic patients with critical stenosis	Not approved, but positive results. Compelling reasons supporting primary (e.g. non-provisional) stenting, to prevent recoil, turbulence and thrombosis, and to reduce stenosis	No published data		Reserved for symptomatic patients who are not PTA candidates	Mild-to-severe symptoms, or asymptomatic with stenosis >80 or 85%. Possible role pre-op before CABG	Moderate-to-severe symptoms
B. Bifurcation and proximal ICA	Experimental but favorable results in recent, non-randomized clinical trials (if performed with stenting)	Investigational. Appropriate for patients not amenable to CEA due to anatomical factors and/or comorbid conditions. Some believe preferred for patients amenable to, but higher risk for CEA	Anecdotal reports of successful use in conjunction with PTA and stent for active or acute lesion	a) Rheolytic thrombectomy (Possis) - anecdotal reports of success in acute carotid thrombosis	Accepted gold standard, for lesions amenable to CEA	Symptomatic or critical asymptomatic stenosis, if CEA not feasible; possibly for high-risk CEA patients	Fulfill NASCET or ACAS criteria

Arterial site and lesion type	Balloon angioplasty (PTA)	Stent	Thrombolysis	Other	Surgery	Percutaneous	Surgery
				b) IIB/IIIA inhibitors — may be useful in carotid stent/PTA. Studies underway c) Emboli protection devices — preliminary experience suggests benefit to capture emboli			
Renal							
A. FMD	Treatment of choice	Not approved. Anecdotal reports for lesions with recoil or restenosis			Reserved for branch stenosis not amenable to PTA	Moderate HTN; accelerated or refractory HTN; renal insufficiency	Accelerated or refractory HTN; not amenable to PTA
B. Atherosclerotic (ostial/nonostial)	Preferred treatment for nonostial lesions. For ostial lesions, incidence of recoil and restenosis high with POBA	Not yet FDA approved, but large body of experience and several prospective trials demonstrating improved results over POBA for ostial lesions	Reserved for acute thrombosis, an infrequent event		Previously accepted standard for ostial disease, although PTA with stent is likely to be equally effective with significantly less risk. Preferred treatment for RAS arising within aortic aneurysm or inaccessible for PTRA/stent	HTN refractory or resistant to med Rx; accelerated HTN; progressive renal dysfunction; CHF; angina. No benefit yet demonstrated when creatinine normal and HTN easily controlled by medical Rx	Same indications for PTRA, when PTRA technically not feasible
Infrarenal and iliac aorta							
A. Stenosis	Treatment of choice	Approved for suboptimal PTA result. Useful for unfavorable lesions. Role of primary stenting controversial but probably improves results and reduces restenosis		Preliminary experience with early endografts not better than bare stent	Reserved for cases of severe diffuse disease deemed inappropriate for PTA/stent	>2/3 category	>3 category

Arterial site and lesion type	Balloon angioplasty (PTA)	Stent	Thrombolysis	Other	Surgery	Percutaneous	Surgery
B. Aneurysm		Stent grafts (covered stents) approved in USA. First line of therapy for high-risk surgical candidates (due to comorbidity), who have anatomically suitable AAA		Coils and occlusion devices required in some instances of AAA stent-grafting	Remains current accepted gold standard for conventional-risk patients	AAA >5 cm diameter and/or rapidly expanding in high-risk surgical patient; AAA causing thromboembolism	AAA >5 cm and/or rapidly expanding; AAA causing thromboembolism
Common femoral	Reserved for patients with severe fibrosis due to previous surgery. Some reports of PTA as first line of therapy in selected patients	Not approved. Flexible stents may be employed under certain salvage situations			Preferred treatment, especially if in association with proximal/distal bypass	>2/3 category	>2/3 category
Profunda femoris	Reserved for cases of severe or limb-threatening ischemia with no good surgical options. Stakes high if SFA occluded already	Not approved. Little experience reported thus far, but anecdotal acute success			Preferred treatment for proximal disease (endarterectomy + patch). Mid/distal vessel not easily accessed	>4 category	>3 category
SFA/popliteal							
A. Stenosis	Treatment of choice for short lesions. Can be utilized in lengthy lesions as initial treatment: long-term results less favorable, but risk < surgery	Not approved. Useful for bail-out indication. Investigation under way using self-expending device. Initial trials with balloon-expandable stents show suboptimal results	Useful only if non-occlusive thrombus present	a) Directional atherectomy may be useful to debulk focal/eccentric stenoses, but no clear-cut long-term improvement over PTA alone	Reserved for cases of diffuse disease deemed inappropriate for PTA or DA	>2/3 category	>3 category

Arterial site and lesion type	Balloon angioplasty (PTA)	Stent	Thrombolysis	Other	Surgery	Percutaneous	Surgery
				b) Rotational atherectomy occasionally useful for calcified plaque c) Trials underway using covered stents			
B. Occlusion	Treatment of choice for short (<7 cm) occlusion	Not approved. Useful for bail-out indication. Investigation under way for occlusion <10 cm	Use highly recommended for recent (<1 month) thrombosis/occlusion. Some operators also prefer for chronic occlusion. May convert short or long occlusion into focal or segmental stenosis, facilitating treatment		Treatment of choice for lengthy (e.g. >10 cm) occlusion		
Infrapopliteal	Appropriate choice for treatment of discrete stenosis or focal occlusion	Not approved. Useful to salvage failed PTA, especially in poor surgical patients	Useful for recent thrombosis or thromboembolism	a) Rotational atherectomy may be useful to debulk calcified lesions b) Trials underway using excimer laser as adjunctive Rx	Treatment of choice for lengthy diffuse disease/long occlusion(s), and not suitable or high-risk for percutaneous Rx	>3/4 category	>4 category

*Indications vary widely depending on risk-benefit ratio of a given procedure in a given patient. These are intended to be general guidelines only.

AAA: Abdominal Aortic Aneurysm; ACAS: Asymptomatic Carotid Artery Study; CABG: Coronary Artery Bypass Graft; CEA: Carotid Endarterectomy; CHF: Congestive Heart Failure; DA: Directional Atherectomy; FMD: Fibromuscular Dysplasia; HTN: Hypertension; ICA: Internal Carotid Artery; NA: Not Applicable; NASCET: North American Symptomatic Carotid Endarterectomy Trial; POBA: Plain Old Balloon Angioplasty; PTA: Percutaneous Transluminal Angioplasty; PTRA: Percutaneous Transluminal Renal Angioplasty; RAS: Renal Artery Stenosis; Rx: Treatment; SFA: Superficial Femoral Artery; TAA: Thoracic Aortic Aneurysm; TIA: Transient Ischemic Attack; VBI: Vertebral Basilar Insufficiency.

References

1. Dotter CT, Judkins MP. Transluminal treatment of arteriosclerotic obstruction. Description of a new technique and a preliminary report of its application. *Circulation* 1964;**30**:654–70.

2. Gruentzig AR. Transluminal dilatation of coronary artery stenosis (letter to editor). *Lancet* 1978;**1**:263.

3. Millaire A, Trinca ZM, Marache P et al. Subclavian angioplasty: immediate and late results in 50 patients. *Cathet Cardiovasc Diagn* 1993;**29**:8–17.

4. Dorros G, Lewin RF, Jamnadas P et al. Peripheral transluminal angioplasty of the subclavian and innominate arteries utilizing the brachial approach: acute outcome and follow-up. *Cathet Cardiovasc Diagn* 1990;**19**:71–6.

5. Dueber C, Klose KJ, Marache PH et al. Percutaneous transluminal angioplasty for occlusion of the subclavian arteries: short- and long-term results. *Cardiovasc Intervent Radiol* 1992;**15**:205–10.

6. Kumar K, Dorros G, Bates CM et al. Primary stent deployment in occlusive subclavian artery disease. *Cathet Cardiovasc Diagn* 1995;**34**:281–5.

7. Ansel GM, Barry SG, Yakubov JS. Primary stenting of symptomatic subclavian artery stenosis. *Circulation* 1996;**94**(Suppl. I):58.

8. Al-Mubarak N, Liu MW, Dean LS et al. Immediate and late outcomes of subclavian artery stenting. *Catheter Cardiovasc Interv* 1999;**46**:169–72.

9. Sullivan TM, Gray BH, Bacharach M et al. Angioplasty and primary stenting of the subclavian, innominate, and common carotid arteries in 83 patients. *J Vasc Surg* 1998;**28**:1059–65.

10. North American Symptomatic Carotid Endarterectomy Trial Collaborators. Beneficial effect of carotid endarterectomy in symptomatic patients with high-grade stenosis. *New Engl J Med* 1991;**325**:445–53.

11. Hobson RW, Weiss DG, Fields WS et al. Efficacy of carotid endarterectomy for asymptomatic carotid stenosis. *N Engl J Med* 1993;**328**(4):221-7.

12. Yadav JS, Roubin GS, King P et al. Angioplasty and stenting for restenosis after carotid endarterectomy. Initial experience. *Stroke* 1996;**27**:2075–9.

13. Vozzi CR, Rodriguez AO, Paolantonio D et al. Extracranial carotid angioplasty and stenting. Initial results and short-term follow-up. *Tex Heart Inst J* 1997;**24**:167–72.

14. Waigand J, Gross CM, Uhlich F et al. Elective stenting of carotid artery stenosis in patients with severe coronary artery disease. *Eur Heart J* 1998;**19**:1365–70.

15. Satler LF, Hoffmann R, Lansky A et al. Carotid stent-assisted angioplasty: preliminary technique, angiography, and intravascular ultrasound observations. *J Invasive Cardiol* 1996;**8**:23–30.

16. Yadav JS, Roubin GS, Iyer S et al. Elective stenting of the extracranial carotid arteries. *Circulation* 1997;**95**:376–81.

17. Wholey MH, Wholey M, Bergeron P. Current global status of carotid artery stent placement. *Cathet Cardiovasc Diagn* 1998;**44**:1–6.

18. Mathur A, Dorros G, Iyer SS et al. Palmaz stent compression in patients following carotid artery stenting. *Cathet Cardiovasc Diagn* 1997;**41**:137–40.

19. Mailloux LU, Bellucci AG, Mossey RT et al. Predictors of survival in patients undergoing dialysis. *Am J Med* 1988;**84**:855–62.

20. Begelman SM, Olin JW. Renal artery stenosis. Curr Treatment Options *Cardiovasc Med* 1999;**1**:55–62.

21. Palmaz JC. The current status of vascular intervention in ischemic nephropathy. *J Vasc Interv Radiol* 1998;**9**:539–43.

22. Klinge J, Mali WP, Puijlaert CB et al. Percutaneous transluminal renal angioplasty: initial and long-term results. *Radiology* 1989;**171**:501–6.

23. Rimmer JM, Gennari FJ. Atherosclerotic renovascular disease and progressive renal failure. *Ann Intern Med* 1993;**118**:712–9.

24. Dormandy JA. Prostanoid drug therapy for peripheral arterial occlusive disease - the European experience. *Vasc Med* 1996;**1**:155–8.

25. Pentecost MJ, Criqui MH, Dorros G. Guidelines for peripheral percutaneous transluminal angioplasty of the abdominal aorta and lower extremity vessels. A statement for health professionals from a special writing group of the councils on cardiovascular radiology, arteriosclerosis, cardio-thoracic and vascular surgery, clinical cardiology, and epidemiology and prevention, the American Heart Association. *Circulation* 1994;**89**:511–31.

26. Mendelsohn FO, Santos RM, Crowley JJ et al. Kissing stents in the aortic bifurcation. *Am Heart J* 1998;**136**:600–5.

27. Tetteroo E, van der Graaf Y, Bosch JL et al. Randomised comparison of primary stent placement versus primary angioplasty followed by selective stent placement in patients with iliac-artery occlusive disease. Dutch Iliac Stent Trial Study Group. *Lancet* 1998;**351**:1153–9.

28. Bosch JL, Hunink MG. Meta-analysis of the results of percutaneous transluminal angioplasty and stent placement for aortoiliac occlusive disease. *Radiology* 1997;**204**:87–96.

29. TASC Working Group. Management of Peripheral Arterial Disease. *J Vasc Surg* 2000;**31**: S1–S296 (Supplement).

30. Perko MJ, Norgaard M, Herzog TM. Unoperated aortic aneurysms: a survey of 170 patients. *Ann Thorac Surg* 1995;**59**:1204–9.

31. Blum U, Voshage G, Beyersdorf F et al. Endoluminal stent-grafts for infrarenal abdominal aneurysms. *N Engl J Med* 1997;**336**:13–20.

32. Parodi JC, Criado FJ, Barone HD et al. Endoluminal aortic aneurysm repair using a balloon-expandable stent-graft device: a progress report. *Ann Vasc Surg* 1994;**8**:523–9.

33. Zarins CK, White RA, Schwarten D et al. AneuRx stent graft versus open surgical repair of abdominal aortic aneurysms: multicenter prospective clinical trial. *J Vasc Surg* 1999;**29**:292–305.

34. Murray JG, Apthorp LA, Wilkins RA. Long-segment (>10 cm) femoropopliteal angioplasty: improved technical success and long-term patency. *Radiology* 1995;**195**:158–62.

35. Gallino A, Mahler F, Probst P et al. Percutaneous transluminal angioplasty of the arteries of the lower limbs: a 5-year follow-up. *Circulation* 1984;**70**:619–23.

36. Capek P, McLean GK, Berkowitz HD. Femoropopliteal angioplasty. Factors influencing long-term success. *Circulation* 1991;**83**:I-70–I-80.

37. Johnston KW. Femoral and popliteal arteries: reanalysis of results of balloon angioplasty. *Radiology* 1992;**183**:767–71.

38. Matsi PJ, Manninen JI, Vanninen RL et al. Femoropopliteal angioplasty in patients with claudication: primary and secondary patency in 140 limbs with 1–2-year follow-up. *Radiology* 1994;**191**:727–33.

39. Isner JM, Pieczek A, Schainfeld R. Clinical evidence of angiogenesis following arterial gene transfer of phVEGF165. *Lancet* 1996;**348**:370–4.

40. Isner JM, Asahara T. Angiogenesis and vasculogenesis as therapeutic strategies for postnatal neovascularization (Perspective). *J Clin Invest* 1999; **103**:1231–6.

41. Isner JM, Walsh K, Rosenfield K et al. Arterial gene therapy for restenosis. *Hum Gene Ther* 1996;**7**:989–1011.

42. Schwarten DE, Cutcliff WB. Arterial occlusive disease below the knee: treatment with percutaneous transluminal angioplasty performed with low-profile catheters and steerable guide wires. *Radiology* 1988;**169**:71–4.

43. Dorros G, Jaff MR, Murphy KJ et al. The acute outcome of tibioperoneal vessel angioplasty in 417 cases with claudication and critical limb ischemia. *Cathet Cardiovasc Diagn* 1998;**45**:251–6.

44. Isner JM, Rosenfield K. Redefining the treatment of peripheral artery disease. Role of percutaneous revascularization. *Circulation* 1993;**88**:1534–57.

45. Henry M, Amor M, Ethevenot G et al. Percutaneous peripheral atherectomy using the rotablator: a single-center experience. *J Endovasc Surg* 1995;**2**:51–66.

46. Isner J, Pieczek A, Rosenfield K. Images in cardiovascular medicine. Untreated gangrene in patients with peripheral artery disease. *Circulation* 1994;**89**:482–3.

47. Baumgartner I, Pieczek A, Manor O. Constitutive expression of phVEGF165 following intramuscular gene transfer promotes collateral vessel development in patients with critical limb ischemia. *Circulation* 1998;**97**:1114–23.

48. Weaver FA, Comerota AJ, Youngblood M et al. Surgical revascularization versus thrombolysis for nonembolic lower extremity native artery occlusions: results of a prospective randomized trial. The STILE investigators. Surgery versus thrombolysis for ischemia of the lower extremity. *J Vasc Surg* 1996;**24**:513–23.